Saying Yes to Life

Saying Yes to Life

Bless you
Elmadine

Evelyn Echos

Evelyn Echols

This book was printed in the United States of America.

Cover Photo by Jennifer Girard.

To order additional copies of this book, contact:
Xlibris Corporation
1-888-795-4274
www.Xlibris.com
Orders@Xlibris.com
17871-ECHO

Contents

Dedication

To my dear brother, Bob, and sister, Gloria
To our son, Bill, and his wife, Jackie

And to our daughter, Susan, and her husband, John

To the many devoted family and friends who supported me through both good and bad times – with special thanks to:

The O'Neill/Conley families

John Meinert

Virginia Rogers

Ron Tully

And my deepest gratitude to Helen Gurley Brown and Walter Cronkite, who encouraged me to write this book.

Introduction

A letter from Walter Cronkite

*E*velyn Echols ranks right up there with the most interesting people I've ever known. By the time you've read this book, I expect that you will agree with me.

She has it all, and has done it exceptionally well. She was a farm girl beauty who sought her fame as a model in New York and reached life's summit as the founder of a travel school that rescued hundreds of girls from the cities' ghettos.

Along the way, she founded a travel agency. Her timing was almost as exquisite as the lady herself. Like a surfer catching the perfect wave, she rode the travel boom as the jet airliner brought once remote places within reach of all. Thanks to her combination of charm and energy, her agency was a great success and she became the intimate of a roster of famous clients. She was one of the few who lasted in the company of the temperamental Joan Crawford. She was a friend of Helen Hayes and Eleanor Roosevelt and . . . but let her tell you about the secrets of her associations with them all.

And, most important of all along the way, she married a good friend of mine from the University of Texas – Dave Echols, a brilliant advertising man. Theirs was a storybook romance that lasted until Dave left us all not so long ago. Their love affair did not just survive their separate careers. It seemed to blossom even more handsomely as, supported by the other, they reached their own heights of success. In their way, Evelyn and Dave pioneered the Twentieth Century American family that proved that a talented, intelligent, sensitive woman could make a career and a home. Evelyn hadn't planned to be that kind of model, but she made it so.

The proof of her success was that, when Rotary International finally chose to let down the barriers and admit women to their organization, Evelyn Echols of Chicago was the first invited to join their ranks.

Her book is a wonderful tale of this wonderful life.

Walter Cronkite

Chapter One

*I*n looking back, I now realize that every experience, good or bad, serves as a Building Block towards our future. My early years were my most trying. The Great Depression was a time when, as an only child, I was often lonely, especially since my parents were working 18 hour days in order to survive, so they had little time for me. Following that were four trying years in Catholic boarding school.

However, having the blessing of living close to nature and the joy of having a great assortment of delightful pets not only sustained me but these years contributed much to my future.

From experience I know that indeed we do learn more from adversity than we do during the good times. Early on, I learned compassion for others and perseverance, especially after completing nurses training when I ventured out into the world.

This was a time with very few available jobs and when applying one never asked about salaries or hours. You were simply delighted just to be employed.

With absolute faith in God, I was able to sustain my-self by being willing to work long hours at very mini-mal wages. My motto was "keep going!"

I have always believed that being born and raised on a farm was one of the greatest blessings in my life. Everyone on a farm has chores and obligations. With that background, I feel I learned early on a sense of responsibility that made a real contribution to my later success in handling life's problems.

Since I was an only child until age 12, my wide variety of pet animals was of great comfort to me. My beautiful duck, Harry, followed me throughout the day. When I began going to school, he sat by the gate and waited for me. When he saw me, he would flutter his wings and quack wildly. My sassy pig, Sarah; my goat, Tallulah, who could jump any fence on the farm; my gentle, loving sheep, Samantha; and my faithful dog, Spot, were also beloved pets. One of the saddest memories in those early years was one morning when I went out to open Harry's little pad. I was not getting my usual noisy greeting. The door was partially open and when I looked in, to my horror, there were just a few white feathers to be seen. A fox had gotten in during the night and I had no more Harry.

When I began school, I received a gift that is every child's dream – my very own pony. His name was Socks, since he was black with four white feet. As many Shetland ponies are, his mood was often unpredict-able. I would ride him the two miles to school, tie his bridle to the saddle and he would happily trot home.

In the afternoon, my parents saddled him up and he would come get me at school. However, if he was in one of his more fractious moods, we would be riding along peacefully and he would suddenly rise up on his back feet, toss me off, and leave me to walk home. It happened more frequently when the weather was cold or rainy. This prompted me to learn to curse like a sailor at an early age. It was only at my father's insistence that I fed this culprit. The impudent look he gave me as I entered the barn would further infuriate me.

I began going to grade school at age five. This was a one-room school where a magnificently dedicated teacher, Mary Migglio, taught 20 children in grades one through eight. Miss Migglio would arrive at school very early in the winter months and by the time we arrived; she would have the potbelly stove burning brightly and would serve us all hot chocolate and cookies. We learned so much from Miss Migglio. One advantage was that while she was conducting classes for the upper grades, we could listen and absorb more than one would think possible. Today, while others are busily getting out their calculators to answer a mathematical problem, I usually come up with the solution much more quickly. For this, I give thanks to Mary Migglio. This was, by far, my greatest educational experience and one which I still benefit from.

I was born exactly one year after my parents were married. Since my mother almost died of uremic poisoning, she was advised not to have any more children. My siblings, Coleman, Kenneth, Robert, and Gloria, did not begin arriving until I was 12 years old. My father and mother were working the family farm that my great-grandparents Brazilla and Lucinda Bassett had settled around 1850 after they arrived from England. At that time, Brazilla stated in a letter to his family back in England that in order to see over the Illinois prairie grass, it was necessary for him to stand on his horse. His reason for settling at Tonica was that it was close to the Illinois River, which would enable him to market his produce in Chicago.

Lucinda must have been a true pioneer woman. She was 37 years old when they arrived at Tonica and delivered five children with the help of an Iroquois squaw in the following few years. The most amazing thing is that four of their five children, including two girls, attended the University of Illinois. One daughter, Irene, later taught English at the Sorbonne in Paris. Ada became a missionary in China. Arthur was a famous concert pianist. In one of his letters home, he stated, "I am at sea on the Hamburg Line, will play for some of the passengers tonight, and will be playing many of the great halls of Europe over the next six months." Herbert Bassett became a professor at Macomb University. My grandfather, Ira Bassett, opted to stay on the farm.

My great aunts and uncles came to the farm for a sabbatical every summer and there is no doubt that they were greatly responsible for my early interest in travel. After dinner, they would gather on the spacious porch and, as I sat quietly in a corner, they would mesmerize me with their conversations about their incredible travel experiences over the past year.

If it were not for the loving kindness and care afforded me by my Grandmother Bassett, my childhood would have been rather dismal. My father was a

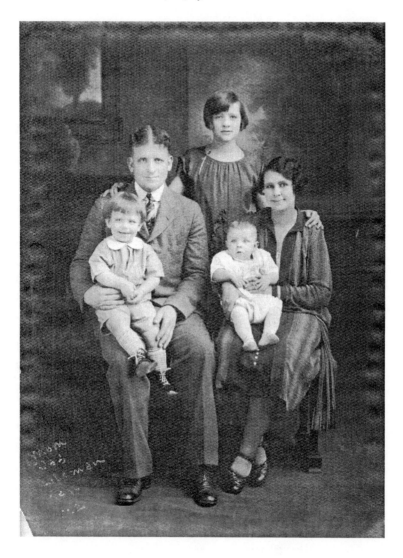

Mom, Dad, Evelyn, Coleman and Kenneth in 1927

man who simply could not show affection. He was also terribly disappointed that I was not a boy, so he called me "Butch" all through my childhood. One thing I am terribly grateful to him for was that each month, when the National Geographic magazine arrived, he would sit me on his lap and read every page to me, explaining in detail those things that I could not comprehend. He was a rebel who had not finished schooling, left home at an early age, and had spent several years working on ranches in Texas. Later, he lived in a hut in northern Michigan all through the cold winter months. On returning home, he met and married my mother – much to the dismay of his family, who were strict Methodists and didn't approve of my Irish Catholic mother.

My mother loved my father without reservation, which I could never understand since he was such a macho character, making every decision in our lives. She was a very pretty, 100-pound woman, who in those early years, loved to dance. However, I recall how often she would spend days crying before he would consent to taking her dancing. His idea of an evening out was to belly up to the local bar with a group of his cronies for hours while my poor mother, her sister, and I waited in the back room until Dad was ready to go home. Every hour or so, he would bring in refreshments for us – the women were not, at that time, permitted in bars.

In my early years, my father and mother were living in a very tiny one-bedroom house, which my dad had built next to the home my grandparents owned. There had been no thought given to adequate closet space so there was no way this house could be kept in order. I presume Dad had thought that now that he was married and had a child, my grandparents might move to a village nearby, enabling them to take over our ancestral home. Fortunately for me, my grandmother insisted that I come and live with them. It was

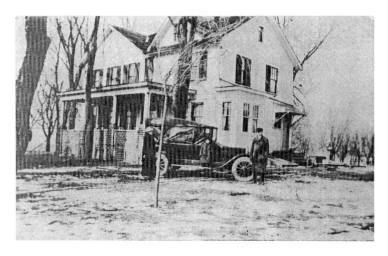

*With my Grandmother and Grandfather Bassett in front
of their home, built in 1870 by my
great-great-grandfather.*

a gloriously happy day at the age of 5 when I moved
my dolls and other belongings to Grandma Bassett's.

This was a lovely house, built by my great-grandfather. The first floor and the staircase all had beautiful
hardwood floors. The kitchen had an alcove built especially to accommodate a huge wood-burning stove.
The built-in oak cabinets also opened into the dining room. The large, sunny bay window in the dining
room was one of the cheeriest places in the house
with Grandma Bassett's six or eight singing canaries
and geranium plants. The table, which had been built
by Brazilla, had built-in extension boards so that when
it was fully opened, it could accommodate 18 diners.
The living room contained built-in library cabinets
on either side of a very functional desk. The upstairs
of the house was comprised of five bedrooms.

At the top of the stairs, there was a bedroom and
living room area, which my grandmother decided

would be mine. I now had a feather bed with a brass headboard covered with a gaily-decorated quilt, which had been made by my grandmother. I had my very own dresser and a fairly large closet. The bedroom opened into this lovely sitting area, which was furnished with two easy chairs, an antique desk, and a commode, which contained a wonderful pink and white china basin and pitcher. On the floor was a bright red, green, and blue Indian rug, and at the windows were white organza tied-back curtains. Another joy about this glorious move was the fact that there was a door leading to the porch rooftop, which was surrounded by tall oak trees. Here, I spent many delightful hours listening to the chirping birds and the rustling trees.

There was only one small problem. In those days, there was no central heating, so when the temperature was 20 or 30 degrees below zero, I was perfectly happy in my wonderfully warm bed with Spot snuggled up as close to me as he could get. "But, oh. . ." in the morning when I had to step out into this frigid room! I soon learned to keep my underwear and stockings under my pillow and get half-dressed while I was still in bed, then complete dressing and make a dash downstairs. The next adventure, of course, was the morning visit to the outdoor john. No wonder so many people in those days took castor oil on a regular basis – we were all constipated. However, I still attribute my incredible immune system and my agility at age 88 to this experience.

In the summer, when the temperature got to be 90 degrees, Spot and I would run out to the farmyard and I would jump, fully clothed, into the cattle's tank of icy water. Spot would join me, and after a few invigorating minutes listening to the hum of the windmill overhead; we would dash out to a cornfield and lie down on the cool black earth. Surrounded by the tall cornstalks that protected us from the sun, Spot and I slept soundly, many times for hours before the dinner bell called us home. On these warm nights, Spot and I often slept out in the yard. When my eyes became acclimated to the wonders of the night, I could see thousands of stars moving through the skies and was, oh, so enchanted as I watched several of them fall during the course of the night. Night sounds in the country were wonderful; especially when the gentle breeze kept the tree leaves making music as they moved to and fro. I loved the sound of the baby birds chirping, an occasional moo coming from the barn, the sad wail of a coyote, and the early morning crow of the roosters as the sun came up over the horizon.

In those early years, my spiritual life revolved around nature. I had an enormous respect – almost awe – for the beauty of nature. And I often wished that instead of spending so much time in church, I could use those precious hours to meditate in the open. I'm saddened when I think how few children of today ever have the opportunity to enjoy the open spaces.

Harvest time was always fun for youngsters. Our neighbors would arrive from miles around to help harvest and bring the grain in from the fields. Their wives would be there to help prepare a gigantic lunch for this hungry group. The huge luncheons would include fried or roasted chickens prepared in large vats, salads, and dozens of desserts, including cakes, pies, brownies, and cookies. My friend, Agnes, and I had the responsibility of keeping the workers supplied with water and lemonade. We would ride our ponies from field to field and have a very merry time. It was pretty exciting to watch the very process of the harvest. The horse drawn reapers were fascinating!

I was raised in two distinct cultures. My father's family led very structured, orderly lives. As Methodists in those years, there were very strict rules of conduct. On Sunday, for example, after church services, we were never allowed to play my grandfather's gramophone or participate in any sports or games. Reading was the order of the day. Then we went to the home of my mother's family, the Colemans, which was two miles away from our home. The main difference was that this Irish American family was more fun. We spent every Sunday and all holidays with the Colemans, with perhaps as many as 20 people. Their family consisted of five boys and three girls. After the quiet of my paternal grandparents' house, the Coleman household was pure bedlam. My grandfather, who danced the jig at all social events, reminded me of Barry Fitzgerald, the famous Irish actor. He was the ne'er-do-well of his family – something his father apparently recognized early on. In his will, my great-grandfather left a farm to each of his children, but the will stipulated that my grandfather could not sell his property. It was to be passed on to his children.

On the Sundays that we went to the Colemans house for lunch, there were assorted aunts and uncles, spouses, cousins, and stray relatives. The rule was that each family brought their own linen napkins, on which they had put their initials in ink. The table seated about 25 people and was covered with a beautiful Irish linen tablecloth. My cousin, Buddy, and I hated to be confined to these interminable meals, and so, whenever we could, we snuck into the pantry, gathered up the makings of a lunch for ourselves, ran down the hill, and hid in some willow trees on the banks of a cool stream that flowed through the Coleman property. Ignoring the urgent calls from the house, we stayed until we were sure the visitors had left and it was safe to come home.

My poor Grandmother Coleman was a slave. It was her efforts that supported the family. She made wonderful butter, cheese, and other dairy products, which my grandfather sold in the nearby town of LaSalle. He was inveterate gambler, and all too often, he left her earnings behind, lost in a poker game in the tavern before he came home. This obviously did not make her a happy camper, so she became very difficult to be around.

I remember the day when, after months of nagging, my grandfather finally bought a new car. As he pulled into the yard, we all gathered around to admire his beautiful REO automobile. Minutes after my grandfather got out of the car, it started to roll downhill, picking up speed until it flipped over, rolling over several times before coming to rest in the stream at the bottom of the hill. My father, trying to console my poor grandmother, told her not to worry because insurance would cover the loss. But then my grandfather sheepishly admitted that he hadn't bought insurance. From then on, it was a rare day that my grandmother failed to mention "that day Ed let the car go into the stream".

Christmas was truly a happy time in my childhood.

My stocking hung over the kitchen stove (since we had no fireplace), waiting for Santa to fill it with nuts, oranges, and apples – rare commodities during the winter months. For many years, I treasured a doll Santa had brought me – it was the joy of my life. I often wonder, when I watch my grandchildren and nieces and nephews surrounded by their expensive toys, if I did not get more joy from that one doll than they receive from all their bounty.

Most of our neighbors were of German descent. There were perhaps two Jewish families in the LaSalle area. I don't believe I ever encountered a black person until I visited Chicago. The Ku Klux Klan was quite prominent in our area. I remember one great adventure when my friends and I hid out in the bushes near our neighbor's farm and watched the ceremonial cross burning, trying to identify our neighbors under their sheets and masks. These people were our neighbors; I had no fear of them, even though we knew that the Klan hated Roman Catholics.

Even in our isolated area, we felt the influence of the gangsters in Chicago. Those were the years of Al Capone and his gang, who were running beer from Chicago to Peoria. Their route took them right through LaSalle County. It was a wide-open town, where gambling was allowed. Capone's gang supplied the beer sold in the local taverns. The reality of the gang wars was brought home to us one Sunday morning. My father, who was not a churchgoer, would drop off my mother and me at the Roman Catholic Church and wait for us at a nearby tavern. One day after Mass, we went to the tavern to meet him and found a large crowd gathered. The tavern owner, who had been buying his beer from another supplier, had had a visit from Capone's men the night before. They had shot up his entire back glass bar, except the area where the owner had been standing at the time. Not surprisingly, he changed beer distributors in a hurry.

About this time, a good friend of my father's, Mike Welter, was elected sheriff of LaSalle County. He gained national fame – and a story in TIME magazine – for stopping Capone's activities in our county. He was utterly fearless. Mike lived with his sister next to the jail in Ottawa, and I would sometimes visit them on the weekends. It fascinated me to go over to the jail and talk to the inmates, who seemed very pleasant. One time, I went with Mike to the Joliet Penitentiary, and the warden took me through the maximum-security area. Those inmates were not so pleasant!

In 1929, after the stock market crash, our lives at the farm began to change. Since my family owned no stock, we were not too concerned until there seemed to be a dramatic decline in the price that wheat, livestock, and corn were bringing in the market. At this time, I was 14 years old and since I was attending a Catholic school in the nearby town of LaSalle, I was only home on weekends and for some time did not notice the subtle changes that were taking place in our lifestyle. I was aware, however, of the fact that my mother was not making her weekly shopping sojourns to town. Most of the food was produced right at home – a lifesaver that people living in metropolitan areas did not experience. Now all of the fruits and vegetables came from our storage bins in the basement where potatoes, apples, and pears were stored. Canning became much more important to us – and oh, how I hated it. My assignment was always the same: to shell peas. It seemed like I would never get to the bottom of the bushel basket. This abundant supply not only got us through the winter months, but also allowed us to help our friends who lived in neighboring towns. My father no longer had regular hired men working on the farm. My mother and father seemed to have no time at all for rest and relaxation. By the summer of 1930, many men were walking through the countryside begging for a day's work. My parents never turned anyone away, and although they couldn't hire them, they would invite them for a meal and allow them to sleep in our barn. It was pathetic because these were not people who were used to asking for charity and were terribly embarrassed by their situation.

My mother had one problem, and that resulted from her upbringing. She was what I call a professional Catholic. She insisted that I go to a Roman Catholic high school. The Great Depression was in full swing and my father could ill afford to send me away to school. But my mother's sister was a nun with the Daughters of Charity, and they had a school in LaSalle. My mother prevailed on them to let me live in the attic with the nuns and attend classes Monday through Friday. Since I was the only boarder, I was alone every day from 4pm on. I was completely miserable. Worse still, I was a country bumpkin, with no experience being around people my own age. I found it impossible to make friends with my more sophisticated classmates. The emotional turmoil did nothing for my grades. I was deeply humiliated in French class when the teacher made fun of my diction in from of all the other students. To this day, although I've traveled in France often, I find it embarrassing to try to speak French.

I had also noticed, when looking out my school window, the long lines of people waiting for their morning rations of bread and coffee, at the church across the street. They would assemble again at around 4pm when the soup kitchens opened. During those days, our winters were much colder than they are today and it was devastating to see those long lines of desperate, innocent victims of the Depression standing patiently, silently in the freezing cold, waiting for just enough food to sustain them through the night. At times, when we were walking down the street in the afternoon, we would recognize someone who was so ashamed of their situation that they would turn and hide their faces. An embarrassing moment happened one day when I recognized Henry Shey in line. He signaled to me not to speak to him. I had known Henry, who repaired our shoes, practically my entire life. I could not believe this usually cheerful, affable man was reduced to having to beg. I grew up quickly in those years and I'm grateful for the experience. This is when I first became aware of social prejudice against those who not so affluent. It was truly shocking to me how some of the nuns at our school pandered to the banker's daughter and gave some of us very little attention.

However, nothing will ever compare to my despair shortly after I began dating at age 17. My first date was an attractive young man, a football player at LaSalle-Peru High School. We met at the counter of our ice cream parlor, where many of us gathered after school.

I was thrilled beyond words when he invited me to go with him to a hot dog roast on the following Saturday night. I wore my relatively new Easter suit that evening. I had a wonderful time and since I had developed quite a crush on Steve, I was enchanted when he invited me to a movie later in the week. Since the suit was my only dressy garment, I added a colorful scarf to it and made a blouse from a piece of fabric I had found in the attic. Steve drove into the yard and when I ran out to meet him, he said to me, "Is that all the clothes you have?" I had not yet gotten into the car, but when I said, "Yes, it is" he turned on the engine and drove off without saying another word. I was not only devastated but also totally humiliated. The only good that came from this ghastly experience was that I lost 10 pounds in the subsequent weeks because I had completely lost my appetite. I made up my mind at that time that this would never happen to me again. So, as soon as I began earning money, I invested most of it in my wardrobe and became something of a clotheshorse.

An exciting new development came about in our area during this period. The gypsies were arriving. I have no idea where they came from or where they were going, but they were scouring the rural areas, living on what they could steal from farms. Word spread quickly when they were in our neighborhood. I was not allowed to go outdoors when they were present, because of my parents' fear that they would kidnap me. However, I found them to be wildly exciting as they came by in their covered wagons, their attire a beautiful array of bright colors.

They seemed to be the only happy people around.

I recall one day my grandmother grabbed her broom and rushed out to chase a young woman who was filling her basket with apples from our orchard. She was spectacularly beautiful, wearing a bright green, off-the-shoulder blouse, with a floor-length, multicolored skirt. She was in the direct light of a very bright sun. Her shiny black hair and her statuesque posture made her a vision to behold. My grandmother's angry demands that she "drop the apples and get out of here" fazed her not one iota. Only when her basket was full did she start walking slowly toward the road, turning back to insolently thank my grandmother for her kindness.

I was particularly happy when the gypsies came by our place late in the afternoon because this meant that they would probably set up camp within a mile of our place. If I kept my bedroom window open, I was enchanted watching their campfire glowing brightly and listening to the beautiful melodies being played on what was probably a zither or possibly a guitar. I would visualize their singing and dancing to this melodic, romantic music. My father and the other men in the neighborhood were not so enchanted by their presence and they never dared go to bed until they had left the area. My father napped on the sofa in the living room, with his shotgun nearby and when we heard a great commotion in the chicken house or the barn doors opening, he would go out and fire skyward to frighten the marauders away. Stealing pigs and chickens seemed to be their night activity while innocently stealing fruits and vegetables from gardens and orchards was a daily activity.

Being an only child for the first 12 years of my life

and having only one girlfriend with a mile and a half was at times very lonely. Therefore, my friendship with Agnes was very important to me. Agnes Baldwin and I had become close friends from the time we began attending school. She had her pony, Hubert, and I had Socks. We would ride our ponies to school, and during the summer spent many days roaming the countryside at will. But our happy times on horseback came to an end during the Depression.

We often attended the auctions held when banks were foreclosing on the farms of our friends and neighbors to offer whatever consolation we could to these poor, desperate families. Their land and all their worldly possessions were sold for sometimes as little as a few thousand dollars. The auction that stands out in my memory was the dreadful day of Agnes' family farm bankruptcy sale, where Hubert was sold for $7.

On this particular day, I noticed that the auctioneer was as ill clad as some of the assembly. As he began asking for bids, I felt that he had been doing this so often that he was completely desensitized and seemed unaware of the tragedy he was initiating. As I observed those around me, the despair was far worse than any funeral I had ever attended. The families – some stoic and others with tears streaming down their faces – the hopeless expressions of the spectators – many wondering if they would be next—and the run-down house, barn and machinery sheds in the background. All of it would have been a perfect subject for an Andrew Wyeth painting.

As Agnes ran out, sobbing hysterically, and kissed the pony goodbye, several men pooled their meager resources and offered to pay the buyer an extra dollar if he would resell Hubert. He refused. As the truck pulled out of the yard, the only sound that could be heard was Agnes' screaming as family and friends tried to console her. This proved to be the most frightening experience of my life up to that date. Not only was I devastated by what I had just witnessed, but I was also wondering how long it would be before I might lose Socks under the same circumstances. When leaving the auction, I mentioned this to my father and he replied in a quivering voice, "Evelyn, I cannot guarantee that this will not happen. I'm doing the very best I can."

I believe my father's reputation for honesty contributed greatly to his being able to borrow enough money from time to time to keep us afloat. There was a small village nearby, Cedar Point, which had been settled by Italian immigrants. The town consisted of five saloons and a grocery store. When my family resources hit rock bottom, I would accompany my father to Joe Cherry's bar in Cedar Point. He would ask Joe if he could possibly lend him $ 200 or $ 300, always giving Joe the exact day he would repay him. This date, of course, would correspond with the time the crops or other farm produce would be ready for sale. Joe's response was always the same: "I have no money but perhaps my neighbors can help." He would then pour my father a beer and me a soft drink and say, "I'll be back in a minute." On returning, he would put the money on the bar. It was always cold – obviously it had been buried in the backyard. Is this how the expression "cold cash" originated?

On the day that a repayment was due to Joe

Cherry, even if the market was low, my father would take his produce to market in order to keep his promise, at times suffering a loss he could ill afford. I'm sure if he had gone to Joe and explained the situation, Joe would have been happy to give him an extension on the loan, but this he simply could not do.

What happened to so many other families like ours? Unfortunately, in those days, there was no welfare, no subsidies, and no government agencies, so for the first time in many people's lives, they had to depend on others. There were no jobs available. Several acquaintances simply could not handle being a burden, took their guns, went behind their barns, and shot themselves – hoping against hope that their families might collect a small pittance from their life insurance. Unfortunately, many times payment was not made in cases of suicide.

But in 1933, President Roosevelt and Congress ordered the banks closed and put an end to the bankruptcy sales. Congress then passed the Work Progress Administration, which hired more than 8 million people in the following years. Most of this work was in construction. Participants built roads, dams and bridges. Another 2 million people were employed in the Civilian Conservation Corps, taking care of government parks, planting trees, and fighting forest fires. Although some felt this was a waste of government money, the President saw it as a better solution than handing out welfare checks.

As the economy improved in the following years, everyone's spirits began to brighten. In celebration, our neighbors got together, cleaned out our barn, and held the first barn dance we had seen in several years. A keg of beer and soft drinks were provided, and as fiddlers played, these happy survivors danced the night away. At the beginning of the war, the economy boomed and many were able to repurchase their farms and life resumed in America, but of course, at a terrible price. Many of the fathers, husbands, and sons who were expected to come home to the family farms did not return, and others came back so physically or mentally disabled that they could never reclaim the lives they had prior to 1941.

About this same time, I transferred to high school in Ottawa, Illinois, where there were about a dozen other boarders. This was even worse than the school I had previously attended because I couldn't go home on weekends. My last two years in high school were equally depressing. I boarded at the Josephinum Academy in Chicago, which another of my aunts had attended before taking the veil. I've always believed that after the Josephinum Academy, boot camp would be a breeze. We got up at 6am everyday, made our beds, dressed and got ready for Mass at 7am. After Mass, we had breakfast, then classes. We were not allowed to talk at mealtimes. A nun read the Bible to us during supper, but we paid little attention to her. Our diet was starchy and I started to put on weight at an alarming rate. Our uniforms were horrible: navy blue serge with rigidly starched white collars and cuffs. The collars chafed our necks until they were bright red. With our uniforms, we had to wear heavy black stockings and wide black sateen bloomers. We nicknamed one of our nuns "Miss Bloomer' because she would stand in the hallway and have us walk up the stairs to make sure we were wearing our bloomers. If, God forbid, we were caught wearing our own underwear, we lost our next weekend leave.

Saturdays were pure torture. In the mornings, after Mass, we had to do our sewing. I remember trying to mend articles that were well beyond repair – a job I hated. I was so slow and inept at the work that I had to spend all of Saturday morning at it. After lunch, the nuns took us for a walk off the school premises. In our stodgy, unglamorous garb, we felt like idiots, and we had to listen to the local boys' rude comments on our appearance. On Sunday, we went to Mass twice. The only excitement we had was when one boarder, the daughter of a local gangster, came back to school after her weekend at home. We'd gather at the window as several cars pulled up and two or three men, obviously ready for any problem, escorted her to the door.

I think I only graduated from the Josephinum because they wanted me out of there as badly as I did. Our final prom was a delight. My mother had managed to scrape up enough money to buy me a white dress for the occasion and the school supplied a corsage. We were taken to the famous Edgewater Beach Hotel on Chicago's North Side for a dinner dance – but naturally, boys were not invited. I didn't care; I was celebrating the fact that I would be gone the next day.

I went home from the Josephinum to a most difficult situation. My mother was suffering from a hip problem and could barely walk. But the poor woman had four children to care for. Shortly after I returned from school, she was operated on, but at that time, hip replacement surgery was unknown and the pain from the surgery only made her condition worse. Money was tight, and because of my mother's problem, I had the enormous responsibility of taking care of my siblings, cooking, and doing the laundry.

Given that I'd barely managed to graduate from high school, I was clearly not a candidate for college. In those days, women went into teaching or nursing. I opted for nursing. At that time, it was on-the-job training with little formal course work. I did my two years of training at St. Mary's Hospital in nearby LaSalle. After six weeks, I was already scrubbing up in surgery. We were on the floor from 7am to 7pm with a two-hour rest during the day. We worked six and a half days a week and were on call for emergencies at night. We had two Sunday afternoons off per month.

One snowy night, a friend and I decided that we needed a break from the monotony, and so we made a date with two interns. The plan called for me to sneak past the supervisor's desk, wearing my uniform. I'd wait under my friend's window and she would throw down our dress clothes. She'd then sneak out and join me outside. We had already made arrangements to change clothes at a friend's house. What we had not planned for was the dozens of utility wires under my friend's window. When she threw the garments down to me, about half of them got caught in the wiring. Despondent, I snuck back into our quarters. The next morning, the supervisor announced the mysterious arrival of a number of garments on the wires outside her window and said that they would stay there until someone claimed them. We had to choose between losing our clothes or losing our Sunday leaves for the foreseeable future. We kept quiet. I lost my winter coat, which I could not afford to re-place, and she lost her only good dress. The supervisor let them wave in the breeze for a week. Each time we passed her window, we were reminded of our folly.

For times past, thank you. For what is to come, YES!

Chapter Two

I have always felt that my life really began with my arrival in New York City on my 21st birthday. However, I now realize how the experiences and hardships of my early years were the building blocks that had prepared me for the challenges I would now face.

Deep down I knew that if I dedicated myself to doing the best job possible I could compete is this competitive market – and I did. When asked what motivated me through those years, I replied, "Because I enjoy eating."

My years in Catholic boarding school had also taught me so much – good manners – deference to others and most important – I was and still am an excellent listener, almost a forgotten virtue in this noisy world of today.

My first venture in travel was not exactly what I had envisioned. One weekend in 1934, my friend, Agnes, and I decided to take a trip to Springfield, Illinois, where we would visit my uncle who was, at that time, a state senator. As was our custom, we never phoned to say we were coming – we thought we'd just drop in.

When the bus arrived in Springfield, we went to my uncle's home. To our horror, we discovered that the house was obviously unoccupied – all the doors were locked. And, to our dismay, no one answered the phone in his office. We now had to find a room for the night. We were very relieved when we saw a "rooms for rent" sign nearby.

A very distinguished, most elegant woman, wearing a black suit with a heavily starched white blouse, met us at the door and invited us in. Since she was the most beautifully turned out woman I had ever seen, I couldn't take my eyes off her, particularly her blond hair swept up in a twist and held in place by a large decorative comb. In later years, I was reminded of how she looked like the actress, Ann Harding. She was statuesque. I was so impressed with her beautifully modulated voice. She seemed to take a very special interest in us. The room where she invited us to sit was like a movie set – lovely antique furniture and an array of spring flowers. Are all rooming houses like this?

She offered us a soft drink and then showed us to a small but pleasant bedroom. We paid her and then, since it was almost 6pm, we went out to eat. On returning, as we went up the stairs, we glanced into the living room and saw that there was a large party going on. There were a great number of beautifully gowned women in the room. The men seemed much older than the young women so we thought it was a party for the local politicians. We would have liked to have sat on the steps and gawked, but since a couple was coming down the stairs, we had to forgo this idea. As we passed the couple, the man gave both of us the type of leer we were not accustomed to seeing.

When we got into our room and closed the door, Agnes whispered to me, "My God, Evelyn, I think we're in a whorehouse." Since I was not really familiar with the terminology, it took me a few minutes for this to sink in. Agnes started crying and was convinced we'd be sold into white slavery. Obviously we couldn't leave now, so we shoved a heavy dresser in front of the door. Our bathroom for the night would be the basin in the room – we certainly could not take a chance on going down the hall to a communal facility.

As we lay on the bed, too frightened to sleep, we made our plans to sneak out at dawn. We listened as the customers were coming up and down the stairs and tried to hear conversations going on outside our door. Once or twice, someone turned the knob on the door, causing our hair to stand on end. About 4am, the noise subsided. We listened carefully to make sure the whole house was now asleep, quietly removed the dresser, grabbed our bags, snuck down the stairs and headed out the back door.

As we passed through the kitchen, though, I noticed a black book near the telephone and grabbed it. Why I did this, I had no idea as we were possibly endangering our lives. As we ran down the street, I showed Agnes the book. She said, "Evelyn, how stupid can you be? That woman will do anything to get that book back." We threw it in a garbage can and

Agnes wisely decided that when we got to the bus station, we would board any bus that would get us out of Springfield.

Fortunately, a 6am bus was coming through, en route to Chicago and would make a stop in Ottawa, not too far from our home. Since we shared our names and addresses – and the fact that my uncle was a state senator – with the lovely madam, every time a stranger came down our road for weeks after, I would run and hide in the basement. However, no reprisal ever came. Perhaps we can thank my uncle.

After I had completed two years of nurses training, I went down to St. Louis, where my mother's sister, Genevieve, a Catholic nun, was an executive at the Catholic hospital there. This was quite an experience because I had left home with only enough money to see me through for two or three days. When I arrived at the hospital, I was met with the unhappy news that Sister Genevieve was on retreat in Kentucky and would not return for several days. In the meantime, no one showed great interest in hiring me.

In desperation, I rented a small room in a boarding house very near the hospital. By the third day, despite my frugal food budget, I ran out of money. I didn't want to stress my parents, so for the first time in my life, I actually went without food for two days. I have no idea how my very nice landlady discovered that I was not eating, but when she brought me a plate full of cold cuts and potato salad, I was so grateful in thanking her, that I broke down crying. She very kindly invited me to have breakfast the next day and I was so ravenously hungry that I ate practically everything in sight.

When Sister Genevieve arrived home, I was immediately employed. When they asked me when I'd like to start, I said I'd be back in an hour with my uniform. This would enable me to be there in time for lunch.

I spent only a short time in St. Louis since an opportunity came up for me to accompany a gentleman who was diagnosed with tuberculosis to the Jewish National Tuberculosis Hospital in Denver. I jumped at the opportunity to see the great West. On arriving there, I accepted a position but shortly thereafter, I was again on the move.

I had always dreamed of visiting New York. From what I had gleaned from magazines and newspapers, this city seemed to me to epitomize everything that was glamorous and exciting. In April 1936, my friend, Elaine, and I had saved up enough money for a trip to New York by car shuttle – the cheapest way we could get there. I wish I could say I had wonderful memories of my trip east. But with our luggage crammed into the back seat and driving straight through the night, it was extremely uncomfortable. By the time we entered the Holland Tunnel, we were loopy with fatigue and barely noticed that we'd arrived in the Big Apple.

Elaine and I got ourselves a hotel room on 63rd and Broadway and slept for almost one entire day. When we'd recovered, we went for a walk down Broadway. It was the day after my 21st birthday. I stood on Broadway, taking it all in, and it felt as though everything I saw was exactly what I had dreamed it to be. All the nostalgic songs and stories about New York in that period barely do the place justice. It really was magic – the frantic rhythm of the streets, the neon lights of Broadway, the fabulous restaurants, celebrities sweeping out of their limousines and into brilliant nightclubs – it was all one could imagine, plus more. We had only planned to stay for a week, but I turned to Elaine and said, " I'm never leaving this city. This is my new home." She agreed but said she'd have to go home to make some arrangements and then return to New York.

But if I was going to stay, I needed to find work immediately. Fortunately, the desk clerk at our hotel very kindly gave me a copy of the Want Ads section of the Sunday New York Times and sure enough, there was a job in a private maternity hospital in an ideal location, at 56th and Lexington. The hospital's owner was an Italian doctor who called each mother-to-be "Rosie". Who Rosie was, I never knew. But her name was shouted up and down the hospital corridors all day, like a delightful mantra: "Push, Rosie, push!"

Someone asked me recently what motivated me to keep moving on. My response was "I grew up during the Great Depression and learned early in life that if you didn't work, you didn't eat. I love to eat!"

One of the most fortunate things that happened to me occurred when I moved into the Barbizon Hotel for Women. This was where almost every unmarried woman who came to New York in the 1930's resided. It was a safe haven in the big city. In later years, I discovered that Grace Kelly had lived there when she first came to New York and had shared a room with Donna Atwater, who became one of my very dearest friends when I later moved to Chicago.

Not surprisingly, men hung around the Barbizon Hotel entrance like vultures, 24 hours a day.

Several of the famous most glamorous models living in the Barbizon Hotel took me under their wings. They were fun, unpretentious working girls with outrageous stage names: Dulcet Tone, Choo Choo Johnson, Dorian Lee (who later owned a highly successful model agency in Paris) and Honey Child Wilder come to mind. They'd been in Manhattan long enough to know the ropes. Choo Choo was probably the most beautiful woman I ever met, and a wonderful friend. She had a delightful sense of humor. She used to love shocking people by saying "I've been giving it away down south before I realized it was worth cash up north".

Lucky for me, these kind worldly girls decided that I needed a complete makeover if I wanted to survive in the big city. They took me down to 7th Avenue to stock up my tiny wardrobe at wholesale prices and then to their own beauty salon, which took a dim view of my unprofessional hairstyle and makeup. By the time they were done with me, I felt transformed – an Alice in Wonderland.

One day, Dulcet and several other models invited me out to a movie. On the way, they stopped by the John Powers Model Agency to pick up their assignments. As I was waiting for them in the reception area, a gentleman walked by and glanced at me. He stopped, turned around and looked at me intently. He asked me whom I was waiting to see, introducing himself as John Powers. I was flabbergasted when he invited me into his office. Smiling, he told me, "You're the most typical Midwesterner I've seen in a long, long time. I think you'd be ideal if you wanted to model for the Montgomery Ward catalogue." And here I thought I was the personification of New York. They took photographs, and I did, in fact, do a good deal of work for the catalogue. But I soon realized that I'd never make it as a top model.

I was very lucky not to be just another Midwesterner, dazzled by the bright lights, but with no connections in New York. My friend, Elaine, had been to New York before and had friends there: the Ellis', a family of prominent attorneys. They were wonderful, friendly people who invited us over to dinner one night and then more-or-less adopted us. After that, we were often invited to their parties and the theater – incredible experiences for an unsophisticated girl from Illinois. Because of their friendship, I was not left on my own when Elaine went back home.

One of the single Ellis brothers, Jack, began inviting me to dinner. He was a sales manager of RKO Pictures at the time, and we went to the movie previews and other social activities in the film world. No newcomer to New York ever catapulted into café society more quickly than I. I didn't have the clothes to keep up with my social life, but my new friends made sure I was always well dressed, lending me things from their own wardrobes.

At the time, Joseph P. Kennedy was president of RKO. I remember one evening at a dinner dance, he and Gloria Swanson were out on the dance floor and as he passed us, he said "Jack, that is a pretty girl you've got with you." He would say the same thing every time we would meet and Gloria, at that point, would very coolly dance him away.

Jack was a man of many gifts, including real talent as a song lyricist. At one time, he was working with Fred Astaire on a number – a venture that allowed me to meet this delightful, charming man on several occasions. The thing that struck me the most about this gentleman was his graciousness and his modesty. If Jack and he were troubled about a lyric, Fred would always defer to Jack, even though I thought Fred's suggestions were usually the better of the two. I was fascinated by the elegance of Fred's wardrobe and went out shopping for new shirts and ties for Jack after our first meeting.

Carmen Lombardo, Guy's brother, also worked with Jack, and so we spent many Saturday evenings at the Roosevelt Hotel, where Guy Lombardo's orchestra played for many years. At that time, this was one of the most popular ballrooms in Manhattan. Long before I danced the night away there, I had listened to the broadcast, "Guy Lombardo and his Royal Canadians coming to you from the beautiful Roosevelt Hotel in New York." My dreams of the past years were coming to life.

Jack also co-wrote songs with Arthur Gershwin, George and Ira's younger brother. Arthur lived with his mother, Rose, at 25 Central Park West. I was enthralled when we first visited Rose's apartment, with its view of Central Park, its elaborate furnishings, and wonderful collection of art. In the living room stood a lovely grand piano. I loved going to her apartment when Jack and Arthur were working together, because George and Ira might be there. They visited their mother often when they were on the East Coast.

Rose was a marvelous character. She loved to play poker and many a night, Jack and Arthur might be busy composing so I would watch the poker game. Many of New York's most illustrious celebrities participated in these frays, including Oscar Levant. One of the most remarkable evenings of my life occurred one evening when George had tired of gaming, went to the piano and invited me to sit with him as he played some of his more recent show tunes. It was amazing to see how he would then simply improvise as he continued to play. I couldn't believe I was sharing a piano bench with one of my idols, George Gershwin. He asked me if I had a favorite number and I replied, "I have a recording of 'April in Paris'". He said "OK, I'll play a rendition just for you." If I had told the folks back home of this experience, I'm sure no one would have believed me. I was rather shy in the presence of George Gershwin and was very flattered by his kindness. I found him to be a very good listener. Ira was much quieter and so our conversations were very brief.

Rose had taken an apparent liking to me and would often call and ask me to join her when she was going shopping. Her favorite designer at the time was Hattie Carnegie. She loved hats and wore them well. She was extremely parsimonious. For example, after a long night of playing poker, she would suggest that we all drive out to Ben Marden's, a noted casino in New Jersey. After losing hundreds of dollars gambling, she would not moan and groan about the money, but about the 25-cent toll on the George Washington Bridge. I found her most amusing and enjoyed many good times with her. However, George's death was an incredible tragedy for Rose and from that time on, she was not the jolly, garrulous person we had known.

Jack and I were now dating steadily. Jack loved the

nightlife, and I have wonderful memories of evenings at El Morocco, where Howard Hughes usually sat with the owner, John Perona, and a bevy of beautiful women at the round table. Our favorite haunts were the Stork Club, where Sherman Billingsley, the owner, gave his favorite guests lovely scarves and perfume. We also enjoyed the Copacabana, with its famous cabaret entertainers, and the 21 Club, probably the most famous restaurant in the United States.

One of my most valued experiences occurred at the Copacabana in the early 40's where I was introduced to the now famous, Julie Wilson, who was then dancing in the chorus at the Copa. I'm so grateful that today, Julie Wilson, is one of my most precious friends.

Jack and I married in 1939 and settled down to a quieter life. I had quit my job at the hospital. The Ellis family, especially Emil, who was a very famous attorney, and his wife, Thelma, included Jack and I in many of their elaborate parties and charity balls. It was fortunate that my good friends had clothes that I could borrow for these events.

One evening that stands out in my mind is when Emil took me to a party at Bernard Baruch's, the multi-million dollar financial wizard. His apartment, overlooking Central Park, had an enormous terrace. I had walked out on the terrace to enjoy the splendor of the evening and suddenly someone behind me twisted me around, and before I knew what was happening, was kissing me. I was so naive and shocked when I discovered it was Bernard Baruch that I blurted, "Mr. Baruch, I am a married woman!" He laughed uproariously. He then said, "Could we have lunch someday soon?" My reply was "I'll check my husband's calendar." This again amused him as he explained to me that my husband wasn't invited. The scenario ended as I quickly walked back into the party.

Sunday morning, December 7, 1941, changed our lives dramatically. We were having lunch at home and shortly thereafter Jack turned on the radio to listen to the baseball game. Suddenly announcements began coming over asking all service people to return to their bases immediately and we learned, to our horror, about what had happened at Pearl Harbor. We were advised to pull down our curtains and to please not use the telephone. Jack and I decided to take a walk and the streets were filled with New Yorkers who could not yet quite grasp the tragedy that had befallen us. We returned to our apartment and spent the rest of that day and sleepless night listening to bulletins from Pearl Harbor.

The next day, Jack went over to volunteer his services as a Civil Defense warden and I went to the American Red Cross to register myself for service. I was assigned to drive a van and my principal assignment was to drive servicemen to their point of embarkation in New Jersey. I would pick the boys up at a locale in lower Manhattan and on the way to New Jersey, would try desperately to keep the conversation on a jovial level.

It was obvious that these young men, who had never before been off the family farm or away from their small-town homes, were now terrorized at the thought of what they would be forced into once they arrived at their base in Europe.

I brought with me a notepad and always asked if

they would sign their names so I could keep in contact with them. Saying goodbye to these young men was heart rendering especially when we got to the pier. Here, bedlam prevailed! The Red Cross workers were serving doughnuts and coffee and there were hundreds of family members; mothers, fathers, wives holding babies, young children – all trying to be brave as they were saying goodbye to their loved ones, possibly for the last time.

After all had embarked, people were waving through their tears as the ship pulled out into the middle of the Hudson River and sailed out toward the Statue of Liberty. Some family members would stand there stoically watching until the ship was completely out of sight. Others left the pier immediately, sobbing. The Red Cross personnel were gathering up their paraphernalia and we all left the pier in a state of utter sadness.

This began to take its toll on me and I realized that only a close communication with God was going to carry me through. I recall stopping at a small neighborhood Catholic Church where I went inside and prayed for well over an hour that God would give me the courage to be able to continue in this work at the Red Cross. I left that church with renewed hope and I found the closer I stayed to my Creator, the more I was able to handle the tragedies we were witnessing on a daily basis.

New Yorkers were completely transformed. As I walked to work, I would pass several newsstands where people were lined up anxiously purchasing the morning newspapers. We had no television at that time and most of our news came through the dailies. Sometimes people reading the casualty lists would begin to cry out and the sophisticated New Yorkers, who never in the past spoke to strangers, would gather round and try to offer solace to this victim of the war. We were all victims because we were all touched one way or another.

In the evenings, I worked as a volunteer at the famous Stage Door Canteen, which had been established by Broadway's most famous stars. Here, young men could come in and spend a few hours trying to forget what lay ahead as they were served sandwiches and soft drinks.

The entire theater community supported the Canteen and it was not unusual to see some of Broadway's brightest lights wearing aprons, making sandwiches, or pouring coffee. My assignment was to act as hostess, greeting young men as they came in the door and making them feel welcome. Some men wanted to talk and some wanted to sit in a quiet corner and communicate with no one.

A wonderful spark occurred after the theaters closed each evening and the stars began to come in and perform. Tallulah Bankhead was a great favorite with her husky voice and her irreverence for the ordinary life. Claudette Colbert, Rex Harrison, Helen Hayes, Bette Davis, Alfred Lunt, and Lynne Fontaine all expended a great deal of time and effort to the Canteen. The Stage Door Canteen enthralled the servicemen and we all prayed that the war would soon be over.

In the early 1940's, we learned, to our grief, that we could not have children. I decided to go back to work and answered an ad for a position at Grant Advertising. The Chicago-based firm was then the second largest international ad agency in the United States. The job at Grant's New York offices involved handling travel arrangements for agency executives. A charming woman, Kathi Norris, interviewed me. (She later became the mother of Koo Stark, the porn star and highly publicized girlfriend of Prince Andrew.) She hired me immediately, and I began what would turn into my career in travel, which lasted my entire lifetime.

My job was tough and I loved it. At that time, Grant had offices throughout South America. It was still wartime, and people had to have a priority designation in order to fly. I spent a great deal of time on the New York/Washington train, en route to meet Mrs. Shipley in the US State Department, the officer who was in charge of airline priorities, visas, and passports. She and I negotiated higher priorities for Grant executives who had been dumped in God-forsaken locations throughout South America. What I did not know at the time was that the State Department was heeding my requests because Grant Advertising offices served as a cover for the FBI and the CIA in Mexico, Brazil and Argentina. A good number of the people I was making bookings for in these areas weren't actually Grant employees, but US government operatives.

Among my other responsibilities was the hiring of clerical and secretarial help. It seems unbelievable that in those days when young women would come to apply for a position, one of their first questions was "Any eligible men here?" If the candidate was someone I wanted to hire, I could truthfully say, "Yes, we're

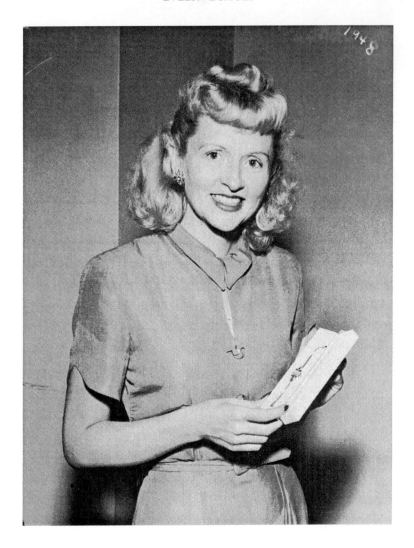

I received my 10 Year Anniversary watch at Grant Advertising.

loaded!" If not, I'd say "No, not really" and they would thank me and leave. Truthfully, I think this was a much better way of meeting your potential life-mate than picking up strangers in bars.

Most of us at Grant were having a perfectly wonderful time. We had luxurious offices in the RCA Building, home of NBC. We were overstaffed and we were losing a great deal of money. Finally, Mr. Grant decided to send his vice-president of international operations, David Echols, to New York to clean house. Within a week, he had fired more than 100 employees, many of them my dear friends. I got a phone call from Mr. Grant's secretary in Chicago who told me that I'd been on the list, but that when Mr. Grant reviewed the list, he refused to have me fired. Apparently this infuriated Mr. Echols, because Mr. Grant was notorious for his rather personal relationships with women employees. Mr. Echols thought I was one of the boss' favorite girlfriends at the time.

What he did not know was that Mr. Grant liked to have me accompany his wife when she was in New York on shopping expeditions, and that I also arranged their cocktail and dinner parties.

Now I was in a truly enviable position. The new manager, whom Mr. Echols appointed before returning to South America, knew that I was untouchable. Life returned to what it had been before the shake-up. But it soon became clear that the new manager was unsuccessful both at getting new accounts and at controlling expenses. Mr. Grant therefore chose Mr. Echols to take over the New York office on a permanent basis. Since he was a handsome 6'2" Texan whose marriage was rumored to be in trouble, this appointment caused much fluttering among the office's single females.

My relationship with the new boss was initially frigid. He told me later that he'd been given a message for me from one of our people in Rio de Janeiro, and it took him a year to get around to delivering it. He hired a new secretary, Petey, who became one of my dearest friends (and still is today). Petey and I were movie buffs and would sometimes spend a weekend seeing as many as three or four pictures together.

In 1949, Petey was about to get married. When I asked her what she'd like as a wedding present, she said she wanted Dave Echols and me to take her to lunch. I said, "No way!" And Mr. Echols reacted the same. Both he and I were extremely reluctant, but she gave us no choice. Dave took us to the 21 Club and spent the first half-hour telling me that he thought I was "the most arrogant little snip" he'd ever encountered. I counterattacked with equal venom, such as "conceited bastard." By the end of the lunch, however, Petey had us on civil terms.

My marriage, meanwhile, was coming apart. Jack had taken to gambling heavily and spent most of his free time at the track. We were spending less and less time together. Shortly after Petey's marriage, I filed for divorce. Although Jack and I stayed good friends for the rest of his life, I was glad the marriage was over.

Shortly after Petey left the company, Dave called and said "I want you to move up to the executive's floor since they can never find you when they needed you." I was having such a marvelous time downstairs with my media friends that I hated to move.

Dave was separated from his wife and living at the New York Athletic Club. He was heavily involved with several women. One day, later that year, he asked me to have lunch with him so that we could work on the itinerary for his forthcoming trip to South Africa. Over lunch, I immediately told him, "If you have any

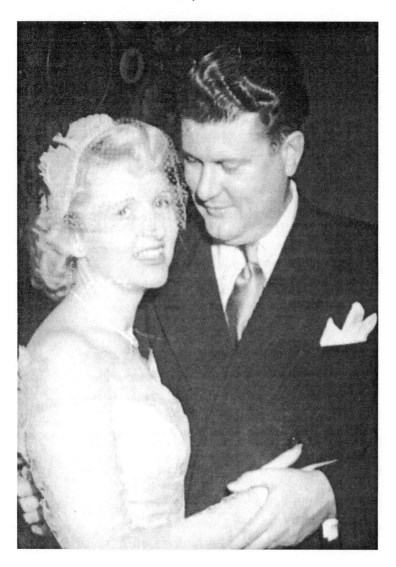

Our wedding day, August 31, 1951.

thought about adding me to your stable of women, just forget it." He laughed loudly and said, "Don't worry. I wouldn't touch you with a 10-foot pole."

Dave went off on his trip, which was a long one,

and after he got back, I found myself in trouble yet again. In his absence, we at Grant's had gotten back into our old habit of celebrating birthdays, engagements, marriages, bar mitzvahs and any other possible excuse for a party during the working hours. One day, a group of us were having a high old time in the art department, celebrating the latest excuse du jour. Mr. Grant, Mr. Echols, and other executives from the office were all supposed to be in Detroit at a meeting with Chrysler. They got back earlier than expected. The door to the art department opened, and there they stood. I was sitting on the top rung of a ladder. Others later said they could never understand how I'd managed to slide past the culprits on the lower rungs and slip through a side door before Mr. Echols began a thunderous harangue. I figured I'd be fired, so I went home, packed my bags, and left for Wisconsin to visit my parents. My father had bought a small resort in the Rhinelander, Wisconsin area and I thought this would be just the opportunity to visit them.

The following Saturday I was listening to the radio in Rhinelander when I heard that a small plane had hit the top floors of the Empire State Building, where Grant was now located. In desperation, I tried to telephone some of our people to question whether any of our employees had been in the office yet. Fortunately, Dave and a group of account executives were not scheduled in the office until noon that day so they had not yet arrived at the building. One of our employees, however, who was already working in the office, was badly hurt when he got on an elevator and the elevator fell.

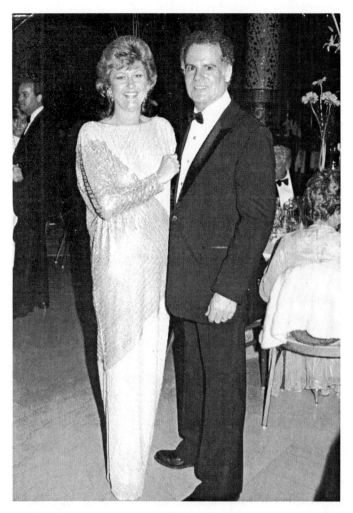

*Our beautiful daughter Susan and her husband,
John O'Donnell.*

To my surprise, a week after that, I received a phone call from Dave's secretary wanting to know when I'd be back at work. I came back sheepishly and resumed my responsibilities.

In 1950, I attended the Annual Grant Christmas

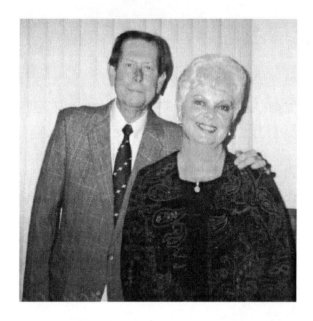

Our Son, Bill, and his wife, Jackie.

party. It was a gala event and I had been dancing for hours. My feet were aching and I had found a quiet corner where I could be by myself for a few minutes. Suddenly Dave came up behind me and said, "You look exhausted, as though you were bored to death. Would you like to go out and have dinner?" I readily agreed. Something magical happened that night and I decided, unbeknownst to him, that someday we'd be married. Shortly thereafter, we were dating. With such a stormy beginning, it was strange to be falling in love. Our engagement stunned Grant Advertising offices. We were married in August 1951, and spent 44 glorious years of wine and roses together, until Dave's death in 1995.

In the first years of our marriage, we unfortunately encountered some serious problems we had not foreseen. David had two wonderful children, Susan and Bill, from his first marriage. However, due to the bitterness of Emmarie, Dave's first wife, we were alienated from the children until they reached maturity. At that time, they came to us and today they are both a great joy in my life. Susan is like the daughter I never had and Bill and I have become especially good friends. Their families are an additional great blessing to me!

For things past, thank you. For things to come, YES!

Chapter Three

*H*ere we ventured into my first experience of living abroad and what an adventure it proved to be! Living under a restrictive brutal dictatorship quickly taught me a greater appreciation for the privileged life I was living as an American citizen.

My memories of Venezuela run the range of emotions and I must admit there were some very hilarious moments.

After we were married, Dave decided that since he didn't want to spend most of his time travelling internationally, he would leave Grant Advertising. He then went to another advertising agency. I also moved on, joining Fugazy Travel Service as an outside representative. In this capacity, it enabled me to have flexible hours and to be able to travel with Dave when he went overseas on business. Then to, I was now eligible for reduced travel benefits which was a great advantage since we spent many weekends in both Bermuda and Jamaica.

About a year after David and I were married, we found a dream apartment overlooking the East River and near the United Nations building. Although it had only one bedroom and was quite small, the enormous terrace captured us, especially since it made a wonderful playground for our two dogs, Sadie – a beautiful cocker spaniel, and Suzy, a mischievous beagle.

On an early May day, I had moved our furniture out on the terrace and had prepared a pitcher of martinis while waiting for Dave. As we sat down, enthralled by our magnificent surroundings, watching boats on the East River, he suddenly turned to me and said, "How would you like to live in Venezuela?" I replied, "That would be about as attractive to me as moving to the Arctic Circle." I thought he was kidding, but he wasn't. Due to his expertise in Latin America, he had been offered what looked like an incredibly fine offer to go to Venezuela where he would be the consultant for Pepsicola Company, which was establishing itself there at that time.

As he waxed such great enthusiasm, I agreed to go. Since they wanted us to move soon, I took on the task of turning my travel business over to a friend. In addition, I had to make all the arrangements for our move because Dave developed pneumonia. It was no easy task dealing with Venezuelan bureaucrats, obtaining the necessary visas and getting permission to bring our dogs into the country. I had managed to obtain passage for us on the W.R. Grace Line so we could at least relax for seven days enroute to our new home.

However, when we got to our cabin on the morning we were to sail, many of our friends were waiting to say good-bye and I was not a happy camper. I felt a premonition that this was not our wisest decision. As we sailed by the Statue of Liberty, I was crying hysterically. One would have thought I was never coming home again.

The second day out at sea, we were having lunch in the dining room when suddenly a crew officer beckoned to the captain who was having lunch. About 15 minutes later, the ship began to roll, dishes crashing all over the dining room. We were told to return to our cabins until further notice. Some of the crewmembers helped us, as it was practically impossible to walk without support. We were told that we were going to the rescue of a freighter. Our ship, which had been heading into the storm with little problem, now had to turn and sail sideways. It didn't take long before I was desperately ill and for the next eight hours I was not really sure whether or not I would opt for the ship to sink. David, who was never subject to seasickness, went up to the captain's bridge with the crew and thoroughly enjoyed the spectacle of the storm from this vantage point. He brought me mashed potatoes and jiggers of vodka, which the doctor recommended I take along with the medications he was prescribing. From my bunk, I noticed Sadie and Suzy were sprawled out on all fours and I decided to join them. The solidarity of the floor did give me some relief. We had finally arrived in the area where the freighter had gone down and joined several other ships in searching for survivors. All ships got into a circle and then one by one crisscrossed over to the other side. Some of the other ships had picked up survivors and we were finally notified to leave the area, as there seemed to be nothing more we could do. Once we turned and resumed our course, I began to feel better and within another day, we were sailing on a calm sea.

When we reached our destination of LaGuaira, our dogs were reluctant to disembark – rightly as it turned out. The port itself was an armed camp, with soldiers toting machine guns everywhere. I tried to get David to get back on board and sail straight to New York, but without success. It took a miserable unpleasant three hours and some healthy bribes to get past the threatening customs officers. Even then, they stole most of our collection of big band and Broadway show recordings, claiming they were "subversive."

A friend, who was later to be a business associate of David's, picked us up at the port and drove us to Caracas. The road was narrow and wound through the mountains. Crosses had been put up all along the route in memory of those who had missed one of the many hazardous curves. (During our stay in Venezuela, a four-lane highway replaced this road.)

Caracas itself is the city of eternal spring. Orchids bloom year round, through the warm days and cool nights. Our friends had rented us a small cottage on the grounds of the Caracas Country Club, where we stayed while we looked for more permanent housing. David would leave very early in the morning. Since offices were closed from noon to 2pm for the siesta, people worked until 7pm. David usually got home well past 8pm. The one friend I had in Caracas was extremely busy and could spend little time with me, and few people used the country club during the week. Sadie, Suzy, and I were left to our own resources. I can honestly say that I have never been more lonely and miserable in my entire life. Finally, I found a lovely-furnished house, available for a short-term lease while its owners were in Europe. After we moved in, life improved. David was making a great many business acquaintances, and we began to entertain at home.

But life under the ruthless dictator Perez Jimenez was extremely depressing. We had been in our new house only a few days when the doorbell at the patio entrance rang. I was home alone. When I opened the door, a man started talking to me in Spanish. I couldn't understand him. When I failed to respond, he reached into his bag, pulled out a pair of scissors, and tried to cut our telephone wires. Frantically, I shoved him out the door and locked it behind him. Within minutes, squad cars arrived at the house and the police demanded that I open the door. Thank God, my neighbor saw what was going on and came to my rescue. My caller had been a representative of the telephone company, trying to collect one month's security deposit from us as new tenants.

Shortly after my run-in with the phone company, we were having a dinner party for some of David's colleagues. One of them had left his car parked, perfectly legally, in front of our house. Another vehicle came around the corner and struck his car. When the police arrived, they arrested our guest – who hadn't even been in the car when it was hit and could in no way be considered responsible for the accident. It took intervention from the American Embassy to find our friend and get him out of jail. Most Venezuelans didn't drive because whenever there was an accident, the driver would end up in jail. I was always extremely nervous when David insisted on driving.

One of my principle problems was finding some way to pass the time. There were good many American families in our neighborhood, and the wives spent much of their time at coffee klatches or afternoon bridge sessions. Neither activity held much appeal for me. After exploring my options, I decided that when Caracas lacked was exclusive men's shop. I would lease a small space and bring from New York some of the better lines of men's accessories. What I didn't know was that wealthy Venezuelan men traveled extensively and did their shopping in Paris, London and New York. So we took my losses and closed shop after a short period.

The poverty in Venezuela was ubiquitous and depressing. A few very rich families owned the country. There was no middle class. Most of the population lived in abject poverty, living in caves and eking out a living any way they could. The problem was compounded by government policy that encouraged the immigration of Italians, to a point of complete oversaturation. Many of these immigrants couldn't find work and roamed the neighborhoods, often with young children in tow, trying to find carpentry or gardening work. Some had beautiful linens with them, treasures that they had brought from home and now offered in exchange for a meal. I am ashamed to say that many of our neighbors took terrible advantage of these desperate people. We hired a number of them to work in our garden and do odd jobs around

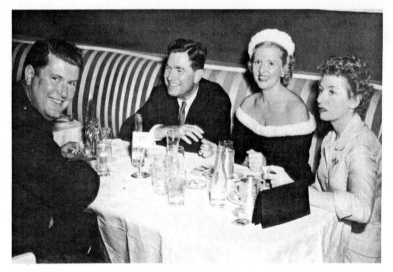

With Patachou, the famed French singer, on her adventure in Venezuela.

the house. David also employed several in his office. One day, we were horrified, on coming home, to find that a young man had hanged himself in our neighbor's yard. We had never seen such terrible poverty.

The opening of the Tomanaco Hotel, owned by Pan American World Airways, was the social event of the year. The famous chanteuse, Patachou, had been engaged for the opening night gala. Her husband and manager, Arthur Lesser, was a man with a fiery disposition. He couldn't communicate in Spanish and was having a terrible time making his wishes known at the hotel. Someone suggested that he get in touch with David for help. That evening, when David and Arthur walked into the pavilion, they were surprised to see television cameras in strategic locations around the stage. Under Pat's contract, television coverage was not permitted. David finally managed to communicate with the station manager, who agreed not to televise the evening's performance.

The next crisis came when Pat walked out on stage and discovered that, because President Jimenez was in the audience, there were hundreds of armed guards around the perimeter of the pavilion with their weapons at the ready. Pat left the stage and found Arthur, watching from the wings. "Arthur, I cannot possibly sing. I'm frightened to death of those armed guards pointing their guns directly at the stage." Escorting her back onstage, Arthur, in his usual sardonic style, reassured her, "Don't worry. As long as you don't hit a wrong note, they won't shoot."

After the performance, Pat and Arthur came back to our house with some friends. Pat made one of her famous omelets. Just as we were sitting down, the phone rang. David answered it. It was Pedro Astrada, head of Venezuela's secret police – an elegant, handsome, soft-spoken man with a notorious reputation for cruelty to prisoners. He wanted to speak to Arthur. When Arthur returned to the table, he told us that he and Pat were invited to Astrada's house – Astrada was having a party and they wanted to meet Pat. Arthur had refused the invitation. We wondered, not surprisingly, whether we might be arrested. It was obvious that Pat and Arthur were being followed – how, otherwise, would Astrada have known they were at our house? Thank God, we heard nothing further about the incident.

The next night's show was to be in the hotel's ballroom, Arthur, who was becoming steadily more and more disillusioned with Venezuela, came into the ballroom and once again found television cameras. In a fury, he pulled the switch, throwing the entire ballroom into darkness. David and I sat laughing hysterically, wondering what the fallout would be from this latest episode. The engineers arrived and, after a long delay that greatly annoyed the audience, got the show going once again. Needless to say, we were somewhat relieved to say goodbye to our friends the next morning.

Xavier Cugat and his band were the next entertainers to arrive at the Tomanaco and their opening night was equally eventful. The President once again appeared. He sent an aide to request one of his favorite songs. Cugat explained that his orchestra couldn't perform this number, since they didn't know the music. Two policemen then escorted Cugat off the stage. We heard later that he had been taken to the police station. Unsurprisingly, the band was delighted to get out of the country.

Life in Venezuela in the 1950's could be hazardous to your health. For example, before the country's Independence Day, the newspapers carried notices warning everyone to be under cover by 7pm because the air force was planning a fly-by over the city and the planes would be shooting live ammunition. Luckily, we saw the notices and barricaded ourselves inside the house – a wise move, since the next morning the yard was full of empty shells and shrapnel.

Our house was on a very busy intersection. Every day, there were at least two or three accidents. Finally, David went down to the police station to ask if a traffic light could be installed. A few days later, as he was leaving the house, he noticed a young boy perched

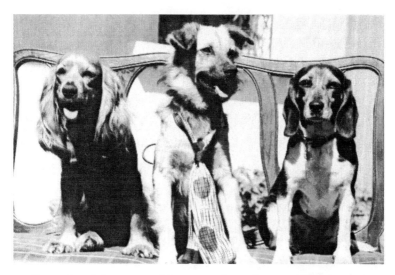

Sam the Man, our Venezuelan dog, with his two
American friends, our Sadie and Suzy.

on a stool at the corner of the street. David walked
over and asked him what he was doing there. "Oh,
Senor, this is my new job. I am the witness."

One day, a stray dog came to our door. He was
starving and bedraggled, but his tail wagged engag-
ingly. Although we worried that he might pass God-
knows-what to Sadie and Suzy, he was such a charmer
that we took him in. We named him Sam. Sam was a
complete joy, and once we got him cleaned up and
fed, he was quite presentable. We kept him to the
patio area of the house away from the other two dogs.
But one night, as we were leaving for the evening, we
found that Sam had gotten upstairs and was having a
romantic interlude with Sadie. Despite our best efforts, we couldn't separate the two dogs. In desperation, David suggested I call the US Embassy for advice. When I explained the problem to one of the

attachés, I got this haughty response—"Madam, put pepper on the male dog's nose." We did, and the problem was solved. David, who had had years of experience with diplomats, always said it was the best advice he'd ever received from an American embassy.

Now that the Tomanaco Hotel was open, it became the favorite hangout for the American colony. The place was always crowded, especially on days when cruise ships put in at LaGuaira. We would gather at the outside bar by the swimming pool and watch in amusement as a steady stream of American tourists, many of them anything but elegantly dressed, dashed through the shops, looking for bargains – foolishness in this high cost country!

Robberies in the area where we Americans lived were a major problem – presumably Venezuelans took better precautions. Shooting in self-defense could lead to a lengthy jail sentence, if the perpetrator survived long enough to make it off your property. Our first encounter with burglars began when I woke up one night to see someone coming into our bedroom. I called out to David, and the intruder ran downstairs and fled the house. We found our dogs sleeping peacefully off a dose of chemical spray. Presumably, we were going to be next. Once we were unconscious, the intruder could have rifled the house for several hours. And what a bonanza he would have had! As usual, clients had paid David in cash, and there was the equivalent of $10,000 in cash lying on the dresser.

The next robbery happened when we were out. The robber was so disgusted by our lack of valuables that he avenged himself by throwing all our clothes on the floor and defecating on them – a common practice at that time. We made a quick trip back to New York to replenish our wardrobes.

We started to feel slightly apprehensive every time we came home from a night out. One evening, I walked out onto our upstairs terrace to fix us both a nightcap. Suddenly, I let out a bloodcurdling scream as I saw a hand coming over the terrace railing. Dave ran out and pulled the man onto the terrace, detaining him while I called the police. The man was begging Dave to release him, saying he couldn't understand why we were picking on him when there were so many professionals working our block.

Finally, our kindly ambassador helped us to get a guard assigned to our house. On his first night on duty, we went to dinner with one of our neighbors, the embassy's military attaché. We came home to find that our next-door neighbor's house had been cleaned out. Apparently, a truck had pulled up in their driveway and thieves had loaded up most of their ground floor furniture and all the silver. When David asked our guard how this could possibly have happened while he was sitting there, the guard answered that he was not paid to guard their house.

Finally, in desperation, we gave up. We were only going to be in Venezuela another few months anyway. So we moved to the security of the Tomanaco Hotel. As we were preparing to leave the house, our friends insisted that we have a garage sale to rid ourselves of the things we wouldn't be taking back to the US. Of course, they used the opportunity to do a little attic-cleaning themselves. On the day of the sale, our garage and lawn were packed with bargains.

About 10am that morning, the wife of the press attaché at the Embassy and I were relaxing up on our terrace. Suddenly an Embassy car came around the corner and Joe, her husband, was calling out to his wife "Ann, Ann, where is my black suit? I'm due in LaGuaira in one hour to meet a delegation and I simply cannot find my black suit." He had tried calling us but our phone was inundated with calls about the sale.

Ann, who was a very tranquil character, said blithely "Well, I'll go down and look. Perhaps I got it mixed up in the clothes I brought over for the sale." Sure enough, it was the only sale we had made all morning. We had sold Joe's good black suit for $10!

Shortly thereafter our very mean macaw had apparently decided there was too much confusion going on in the house for his taste, had climbed off his perch, and had jumped out into the street. He was now about ½ block away from the house enjoying his freedom and had no intention of being recaptured. We finally had to get a huge cage from the Animal Welfare Organization and it took the assistance of several police officers to finally bring him home.

During this time with the doors constantly being opened, our dogs, Sadie and Suzy decided they would join in the merriment. When I realized they had escaped, I was frantic because the procedure for eliminating rabies in Venezuela was to come through the neighborhoods and throw poison meats on our lawns.

Ann called over to the Embassy and now there were about 3 Embassy cars circling the blocks, calling out to Sadie and Suzy. Finally, we located them and thank God, they must not have been too hungry and they were well and hearty.

That night we were so glad to finally have the garage sale day over. After we totaled up the cost of drinks and food for the day, this garage sale proved to be one of my least successful business ventures.

Six months later, after a series of farewell parties, we flew back to New York. I still remember how absolutely delighted we were as the plane circled and started to head north.

We had to leave poor Sam behind. Sadie and Suzy were coming back with us, but we couldn't bring our adopted mutt. Fortunately, our next-door neighbors, whom Sam was very happy with, adopted him. We were crushed when, 10 days later, we got a letter saying that Sam had run away. We had little hope for Sam's survival.

Three months later, David had to back to Venezuela for a Pepsicola meeting. As he pulled up at the building, he heard what sounded almost like a human scream. Sam leapt through the open car window and landed on David's lap, wild with joy. Apparently, Sam had tracked David's car to the Pepsicola headquarters the day before our departure. David said later that one of the most touching experiences in his life was holding this dirty, emaciated animal, who was showering him with dog kisses. He could only imagine how much Sam had suffered over those months, without ever giving up hope that we would return. His survival was a miracle.

Luckily, the woman who operated the Christian Dior shop in the Tomanaco Hotel had known Sam from visiting our home in Venezuela and had found him charming. She agreed to adopt him. When David last saw Sam, he was splendidly turned out in a jeweled collar and a very fancy leash on his penthouse terrace.

For things past, thanks. For things to come . . . . YES!

Chapter Four

*N*ow came one of the greatest challenges I would ever experience – when I became an entrepreneurial travel agency owner. Needless to say in those years, a woman entrepreneur did not receive much attention or support. The airlines were most reluctant to supply me with ticket stock and my landlord would only agree to a six-month lease. He was sure my demise would happen in a short period of time. Added to my problems was the fact that I had determined that this would be a commercial agency rather than a leisure vacation agency. What audacity to believe I could compete with the giants – American Express, Thomas Cook and the other huge commercial agencies. But I did – and with great success!

I now felt I could sing Frank Sinatra's line from "New York, New York". "If you can make it here, you make it anywhere!"

In 1954, after returning to New York from Venezuela, David and I decided that this might be the right time for me to open my own travel agency. Unfortunately, we made a poor choice when we purchased an existing agency whose client list had been grossly exaggerated and was by no means the lucrative business we had expected. We had agreed that my agency, International Travel Service, would specialize in commercial accounts – a difficult route for a woman entrepreneur, I can tell you! At first, it was a scramble to find business. One of my first accounts was the Relin Public Relations Firm. They did a minimal amount of international travel, and we could only charge a five percent commission on domestic flights, so the account generated very little in the way of revenue. Nonetheless, I had to put in long hours to get space for Mr. Relin on TWA's coast-to-coast flight, which offered berths. It was the only airline to do so, making competition for these coveted spots fierce. You might ask why I bothered. My rationale was that Relin represented Pepsicola. If I gave the smaller firm first-rate service, they might open some important doors for me.

And that indeed was exactly what happed. One happy day, I got a phone call from Mr. Relin saying that Alfred Steele, chairman of the Pepsicola Company was marrying Joan Crawford, the famous movie star. They wanted to honeymoon on the luxury liner, *SS United States*, which was sailing for Southampton in about three weeks time. Despite their best efforts, the travel departments of Pepsi, Columbia Pictures, and NBC had been unable to get them in one of the four suites they would accept. Adrenaline pumping, I grabbed a cab and took off for the U.S. Lines office in lower Manhattan. I found, to my discouragement,

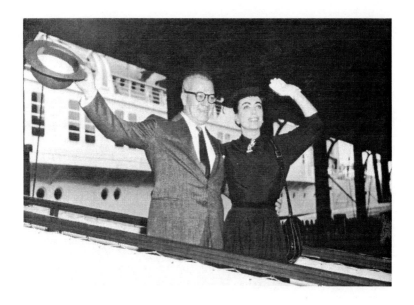

*Al Steele and Joan Crawford sailing off on their
honeymoon.*

that not only was the entire ship booked on full deposit, but also that there was a long waiting list on
which Al Steele's name was about 25th on the list. I
gently persuaded the steamship company's public
relations department to jump Steele's name to first
place on the waiting list – since the PR generated by
having Joan Crawford on board would be most advantageous to the company.

It was now approximately ten days before sailing
time and the situation looked hopeless. However, I
continued to make my daily visit to the U.S. Lines office and one day, a suite was cancelled and I asked for
an option. My friends in the booking office scoffed at
the notion that I could offer this lesser suite to the
Steele's; obviously they would not accept it. What my
friends didn't know was that during my daily visits, I

had managed to note the names, addresses, and phone numbers of the four clients who were holding the U 80-90 suites – the best on the ship. I sped back to the office – names and numbers in hand – and grabbed the phone. Unfortunately, I'd forgotten that it was three hours earlier in Wyoming. I woke this poor gentleman up, blurting out, "Mr. Edwards, you are standing in the way of my whole career." The kind man laughed and said, "How can this be since I don't even know you?" I explained my problem and made him an offer. The suite I had the option on was nowhere near as luxurious as the one he was holding, but if he would agree to switch with me, I would gladly pay his passage. This would be a small investment in what I hoped would enhance my potential with Pepsi. He shocked me beyond belief when he said, nonchalantly, "I really don't care where I am as long as you guarantee me that I will be comfortable and promise to introduce me to Joan Crawford." This, I assured him, could be arranged!

Breathlessly, I called the U.S. Lines and pleaded with them to call Mr. Edwards immediately for a confirmation. I wanted them to get to him before he had a chance to become fully awake. They called me back a few minutes later and congratulated me on my coup. I then called Mr. Steele who refused to believe me until I told him I would be coming immediately to pick up a deposit. When I got to his office, I suggested he call the U.S. Line for confirmation. He did so, put down the phone and leaned back in his chair. With the wonderfully infectious Al Steele laugh, he said "Okay, missy, you tell me how you managed to steal this space from all the big ho ho's that were working on it for me." I explained what I had done and we had a good chuckle. He called his secretary into the office to dictate a letter to the Pepsi travel department, instructing them that from that date on, they were to book all their reservations through Evelyn Echols. He added that if I was astute enough to outsmart them, I deserved the account. Of course, this didn't endear me to the people in Pepsi's travel department, and for some time our relationship was not exactly friendly.

I had not met Joan Crawford until the day of sailing and, needless to say, I was rather apprehensive. I arrived at the ship very early to be sure that all was ready for the sailing party that would be seeing the Steele's off. The beauty of the suite was enhanced by the many magnificent floral arrangements from friends. The 21 Club had sent a huge container of caviar, which was placed in the center of the living room cocktail table and surrounded by buckets of iced champagne and vodka. Joan and Al arrived and I was gratified to see how gracious and warm she was in thanking me. I reminded her of our promise to have Mr. Edwards meet her and she immediately asked to have him brought to the suite. He was enchanted by her charm. As the whistle sounded the time for visitors to leave the ship, we were all having such a good time that we were reluctant to depart. We all stood on the pier waving to the newlyweds as the tugs began to push the ship out into the harbor.

I went back to my office feeling that I would have no problem in future negotiations with Joan. This proved to be true as Joan and Al were largely responsible for the success of my agency. Through their business connections and personal acquaintances, I was able to secure varied accounts. What I did not know was that the real work was yet to come!

The Steele's travel arrangements were often most unusual. On one occasion, Al called from Rome to say he would appreciate it if, on their flight to Nairobi the next day, I could arrange to have the seats in the plane's first class section removed and two beds installed. They also wanted to have the section curtained off, to ensure complete privacy. Al explained that he was exhausted and had to make an important speech on their arrival. After a little thought, I decided that I'd better go straight to the top with this one, so I called the chairman of British Overseas Airlines. I said I was calling on behalf of the chairman of the Pepsi Company, and when Sir William came on the line, I made it clear up front that cost was no object in what we were requesting. I outlined in detail what the Steele's wanted and at the end of my monologue, there was what seemed like an interminable transatlantic silence. At last, Sir William spoke and with true British humor inquired, "Mrs. Echols, do you happen to have any preferences for the color of the curtain?" The plane arrived in Rome, altered to meet our specifications, and the Steeles were able to rest comfortably on their way to Nairobi. I've often wondered what the Pepsi stockholders would have said if they had seen the size of the five-figure check we wrote to the airline.

All of that, however, was a walk in the park.

Where does an 800-pound gorilla sit? Anywhere she wants. This was Joan Crawford's philosophy of life. She was going to have her way. One night, my husband and I went out to dinner with the Steeles, where Joan insisted on ordering the meal for her guests. She decided we were all to have the duck with chocolate sauce. David and Al refused at first, but eventually gave in. I refused outright, which did not ingratiate me to her, but the next day, I was the only one who was not sick.

Joan's eyes said it all. Anyone who has seen one of her films can understand that. When she was angry, she had a glare that could terrify a tiger, but a moment later, those same eyes could knock you over with her charm, where you were a fan or a Pepsi bottler. Her hatreds were legendary. We attended a screening of "Whatever Happened to Baby Jane?" in which Joan starred with Bette Davis, whom she especially detested. Joan was extremely uptight at the screening and tried to calm herself by knitting. The clicking of the needles went faster and faster as the movie progressed, much to the disturbance of everyone around her. At one point, I whispered to David that the makeup department had done a wonderful job of making Bette Davis (who was three years older than Joan) look like an old hag. Joan, never missing a stitch, said, "Oh no dear, that's all Bette." Given her temper, I was doubly glad she never had a single harsh or mean word to say to me.

Joan was such a perfectionist that it could take her two or three hours to get ready to cross the street to visit a neighbor. At the time when I was working with her, she was in her fifties but had kept her youthful figure. This was due in part to a daily massage she underwent that was so rigorous; few people other than professional athletes could have withstood it. She could put away a tremendous amount of vodka without gaining weight. There was always an extra pair of hose in her handbag because heaven forbid anyone should catch her with a run in her stocking. In contrast, Al was a laid back, completely relaxed man who, until he married Joan, enjoyed life to the fullest. He loved people and was very popular with all the employees at Pepsi. This was a complete contrast to Joan's hyper personality.

They lived in a magnificent vintage duplex on upper 5th Avenue, overlooking Central Park and the Metropolitan Museum. She kept several pairs of slippers near the door to give their guests, who were required to remove their shoes in order to protect the snow-white carpet. Beautiful pieces of furniture were covered in plastic, making a magnificent home look positively sterile. Joan's closets were fascinating. Meticulously laid out, they held fully coordinated outfits in military formation and all the garments were on padded satin hangers. No wire hangers were permitted, just as her daughter, Christina, said in "Mommie Dearest". She had a separate custom-made cedar closet to house her many furs.

On many occasions, after I had met with Al and other Pepsi executives who would be going on a trip, Joan would call me and ask me to bring the itinerary to the apartment and we would have breakfast together. After greeting me, we would proceed to the kitchen where she would don a perfectly starched apron. I was amazed at how beautiful her face was, even without makeup. However, I would watch her, noting how close to the surface emotions ran. The kitchen, with windows overlooking the park, was one that you would expect to see in architectural magazines and needless to say, everything was in perfect order. We would sit on stools around the kitchen island that was set with her lovely linen placemats and napkins. When she was scrambling eggs with her wire spatula, she beat the eggs with such vigor that it sometimes made me laugh. I attributed her aggression to the fact that she was annoyed by certain plans in the itinerary. If I saw her jaw begin to set in the famous Crawford manner, I knew that she would soon be picking up the phone to attempt to convince Al to make changes. Usually she was unsuccessful, which did not make her a happy camper.

She needed everything to be, in one of her favorite words, perfect. When this ambition was thwarted, her tension grew to an almost unbearable level. Often times, things would get so tense during these sessions that I would have to take a two mile walk just to calm myself down. Joan demanded perfection not only for herself but also for those around her. One day I arrived at the apartment directly from the airport early in the morning without taking the time to pull myself together. When Joan opened the door, she looked at me and said "Well, what the hell happened to you?" I explained to her that I had flown in from the west coast on a night owl flight and was exhausted. Her reply was, "That's no excuse. You look like an unmade bed and I hope you have the good sense to never allow David to see you looking like this." She then said, "I want you to repeat after me 'from this day forward, I will never again leave the house until I know that I look so beautiful that anyone passing me in the street will think I'm on my way to a romantic interlude' ".

When Joan traveled, depending on the length of

the trip, her luggage could consist of anywhere between 10 to 25 large suitcases, hatboxes, a cosmetic case, and a large jewelry case, which she had to carry by hand. Needless to say, I had to be extremely careful not to make any mistakes when handling the Steele's luggage. Airline special services would have to be notified of their arrival at the airport so that someone would put them in the VIP room immediately and make sure they were pre-boarded. If Joan's two French poodles were coming along, a special seat had to be reserved for them. Arrangements also had to be made for airline personnel to meet them at their destination and escort them directly to their limo. God help everyone involved, especially myself, if when Joan entered her hotel suite, she did not find a supply of Smirnoff vodka and Pepsi, vases of fresh flowers throughout the entire suite, and an ironing board set up in her bedroom. Despite her aristocratic bearing and demands, she never totally abandoned her hardscrabble roots. One day, I arrived at the Ambassador East Hotel in Chicago shortly after the Steele's arrival and found Joan, in her travel clothes, on her hands and knees, scrubbing the bathroom floor.

Although Joan was never cruel to me, I had the opportunity to see how devastatingly cold she could become in an instant. She would be standing at a party talking to a person, charming smile and all, and then turn to me and say, "This is the dullest creature I've ever encountered in my life," or "Get me the hell out of here." Joan had little patience with people but loved animals. I came over one day when she was working at her desk. We went to the kitchen for lunch, and upon returning to her office, we discovered that Mr. Pepsi, her poodle, had just wee-weed all over dozens of her papers. I assumed that this would be his last day on earth, instead Joan simply scolded him briefly and returned him to his playpen.

Joan and Al's marriage was contentious from the outset, and it did not take long for this news to spread throughout the company. Edie Davis, Nancy Reagan's mother, told me once about a dinner that the Steeles' had invited her and Dr. Davis to at Romanoff's in Hollywood where, as Edie said, "Joan was being an extreme bitch all night." Al finally excused himself under the pretense of going to the men's room, and after awaiting his return for quite some time, the guests discovered that he had actually departed from the restaurant, gone to the airport, and flown back to New York. He removed his belongings from the apartment and moved in with a friend before Joan returned. After a great deal of buttering up by Joan, they reconciled and he returned to the apartment.

One Christmas, they decided to take Joan's four adopted children, Christina, Christopher and the twins, Cynthia and Cathy, to St. Moritz, Switzerland. I was there to see them off and could feel the tension brewing like a storm. Her jaw was set tight like it was wired in place, and apparently, nothing changed in the Alps and it was a miserable vacation for all. I was never witness to any of the abuses reported so scathingly in Christina's book "Mommie Dearest" or any of the other rumors that have been reported. Her children lived apart from her, even the young twins, who were in a hotel across the street with their governess. One day, we were having lunch upstairs at 21

– the twins Cindy and Cathy were with us. I was facing the stairs and said, "Oh, here comes Cary Grant." The girls turned around to see him. Joan was furious and was carrying on about how rude it was to stare at people. Trying to alleviate the situation, I laughingly said, "Well, I'm sorry, Joan, but I'm staring." This did not help much and did not stop her from haranguing the girls.

I could never account for some of Joan's decisions. For example, one time I booked the twins and their governess on the French liner, *the Flandre*, to sail to Europe in July of 1956. Joan had ordered the nanny to confine the children to their cabin for the entire voyage. Shortly after leaving New York, however, news came that the luxurious Italian ocean liner, *the Andrea Dorian*, had collided with another ship and was sinking. *The Flandre*, picked up the distress signal, went to rescue the survivors and return to New York. Due to the trauma the children had just experienced, and what I presume to be their fright to being locked inside the ship's cabin, I asked the nanny to ignore Joan's quarantine edict. She complied.

In 1959, Joan and Al asked me to book them a flight to Jamaica. She then invited David and me for cocktails at their apartment the night before the flight. I arrived early and was reading a magazine on the first floor when Al came into the room. He looked extremely exhausted and unhappy at first, but immediately became the familiar cheery Al I knew and loved as soon as he saw me. Joan came downstairs a few minutes later and began serving caviar and champagne. She said it was a celebration of their upcoming trip. Al said he did not feel well and only wanted a glass of milk. Dave and I watched for at least the next

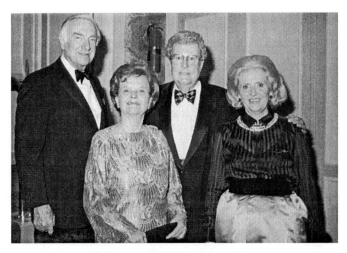

Betsy and Walter Cronkite.

15 minutes as Joan attempted to persuade Al to try some of her elegant offerings. Al refused, upsetting Joan who rang the bell to have the maid bring Al his milk. That night, as we left her apartment and drove home, both David and I were completely depressed. We thought that Al would not survive much longer living with Joan since her extravagances had caused him to fall into debt and her constant demands were taking a dreadful toll.

The next morning was beautiful and David took advantage of it by sitting out on the lawn as I made breakfast. We were on the Jersey shore, where we summered in those years. The phone rang. I picked it up and was surprised to hear Joan's voice because she and Al were already due at Kennedy Airport. In the calmest, most unemotional voice, she said, "Al died last night." I asked her to repeat what she said, either because I didn't believe I heard her correctly or because I didn't want to believe it. "Al died last night. Come on in to the apartment." I was in utter shock, as was David, because Al was not only a client but had become a cherished friend of ours. When we arrived at the apartment, a number of friends and Pepsi executives were already there. Joan played the role of hostess perfectly as though she were giving a lovely party. She never shed a tear and entertained her guests while simultaneously making funeral arrangements. After Al's death, Joan, despite considerable opposition from several executives, was again appointed to the Pepsi board and continued to act as a company spokesperson. However, her lavish travels were considerably curtailed, so as time went on, I saw less and less of her.

The last time David and I saw Joan was in 1977 when she agreed to have dinner with us along with Mitchell and Elsa Cox. Mitchell, the former vice president of Pepsi's public relations department and a close friend of the Steles, was one of the few people Joan trusted implicitly. The plan was to go to Joan's place for cocktails and then go out to dinner. Joan's finances were not what they had previously been, and she was no longer living on 5th Avenue. She now resided on East 69th Street in a more modest five-room apartment. When Joan opened the door, we were surprised to see that she just came out of the shower and was wearing a robe and had a towel wrapped around her head. Even with no makeup and having just crossed the 70-year mark, she was still strikingly beautiful. She said she was sick and could not go out with us, but she still had us in for a round of drinks. By this point, she was practically a recluse and we learned later that she had been afraid to leave her home. I wrote to her from time to time but received no reply. Upon returning from a European trip in

1977, we received word that Joan had passed away from an apparent heart attack.

She and Al left an incredible scrapbook of memories. Those of Al were happy ones; those of Joan were a strange mixture, mostly sad. She had led a tormented life and was a deeply private person in many ways. After Al died, I told her that I had never seen her cry. She said, "I learned a long time ago to cry alone." Her response revealed her isolation and saddened me.

Although clients like Joan Crawford demanded a great deal of personal service from me, I was blessed with a superb staff. My number one asset was Henry, our delivery boy. Henry had come to us one day when we were in desperation. Our regular employee had not shown up and there were dozens of tickets to be delivered. Henry came in to apply for a job and we hired him on the spot. Henry was ahead of his time, not only was he disheveled, but he was also wearing his hair down to his shoulders – all of this in the mid-fifties! He also spoke the language of the ghetto, his home. After two or three days, we realized that our tickets had never been delivered so quickly, and told him that he was obtaining visas at various consulate offices in record time. I called him into my office and told him that we wanted to keep him, but he had to get a haircut and acquire more conservative clothing. Henry said, "Jeez, Mrs. Echols, if I walk back into my neighborhood looking like that, I'd get killed." But to keep his job, he succumbed to a haircut and went shopping with my husband. Yes, sure enough, he did get beaten up when he went back to his neighborhood, but David solved this problem brilliantly. Since we were giving so much business to a particular limousine company, we were given complimentary limo service whenever we needed it. David put Henry in the back seat of this luxurious car, told the driver to take him home, and to circle the neighborhood until all the pool halls had emptied out and everyone was on the street to see Henry's auspicious arrival. The chauffeur's account of this episode was hilarious. Henry had brought a big cigar and was sitting in the back seat smoking. Once a good crowd had gathered, the chauffeur drove up to Henry's house and, with due ceremony, opened the back door of the car and tipped his hat. Henry stepped forth with great aplomb and said, "Thank you, Tony. I'll see you in the morning at 9am." Dave's plan was a complete success, and from that day forward, Henry was a neighborhood celebrity.

Henry could charm his way through any situation. When delivering tickets, he refused to leave them with secretaries and insisted on meeting the person to whom they were directed. General Sarnoff, chairman of NBC at the time, once spent 20 minutes explaining to Henry the responsibilities of CEO. Al Steele invited him to join him for lunch if he was eating at his desk. I had taken Henry to the Steele's sailing party and Joan had graciously posed for a picture with him – something that only increased his cachet. One day, when he was delivering tickets to Dinah Shore, he was gone for an exceptionally long time – he said he'd been invited for tea and could hardly refuse.

Henry made all of our bank deposits at Chase Manhattan, and in typical fashion went directly to a bank officer rather than making his deposits with a teller. The bank employees were so intrigued by him that if he failed to show up at the bank, they would call to find out what happened. Henry looked after me every hour of the day and worried about the hours I kept and whether I was eating properly. One morning, I came downstairs at 5am on my way to Idlewild Airport to greet some NBC executives in customs and found Henry asleep on the sofa in the lobby. He did not want me to go to the airport alone. Henry later told me that the day I hired him he had a penknife in his pocket and had planned to rob me. I've often thought, looking back, that I'd rather have poor, uneducated Henry working for me instead of some of the MBA's I have since hired. When we were moving back to Chicago, the saddest part of selling my agency was saying goodbye to Henry. We stayed in touch, however, and we were deeply amused to find that the Chase Manhattan Bank had hired him.

In 1956, I got a call from a senior vice president of NBC who was originally from Philadelphia and a friend of Grace Kelly's. He said that he needed help in making the arrangements for the entourage going to Miss Kelly's wedding to Prince Rainier. The NBC travel department was having trouble with the bookings, and he wanted to refer this business to me. Of course, I was delighted.

Miss Kelly's original plan was to fly to Monaco, but she later decided that she would like a respite before the weeklong wedding so she chose to sail on the *SS Constitution*. As soon as she made this change, our phones began to ring from early morning until midnight with wedding guests fighting desperately for cabins on the ship. In order to accommodate this demand, I had to hire extra staff, but even so, this assignment turned into a tremendous task. We did manage to book some cabins but not nearly the number we were asked to acquire. For example, Jinx Falkenberg, then a famous television talk show star, was booked in a single cabin. A woman called, identified herself as Jinx's companion, and told us that Jinx wanted to change the reservation to a double cabin. We spent a good deal of time and effort making the change only to find that Jinx had no idea who this woman was and she demanded that we get her original reservation reinstated immediately.

The night before the wedding, all our passengers were either in Monaco or on their way, except for Ike Levy, on of the founders of CBS and his wife. They were to leave on Air France at 7pm. David and I had decided that I needed a few days rest after all the hectic arrangements, so we had booked a flight to Bermuda at 8pm that same evening. We checked in at Idlewild Airport and had some time to spare before our flight. I decided to go to the Air France counter and bid adieu to the Levys – only to find they had not yet arrived. At 7pm, Air France said they could not delay their departure more than 10 minutes, so at 7:10pm, I watched in dismay as the doors closed and the plane taxied away from the gate. Since I knew Mrs. Levy was carrying an important dress for Miss Kelly, I was doubly disturbed. Just as I was walking away from the Air France counter, a limousine pulled up and the Levys emerged and sauntered towards where I was standing. Hysteria took over when they learned they had missed the last flight to Monaco because of their confusion over daylight saving time. Thanks to the accommodating Air France staff, we discovered that Pan Am had a flight departing for Paris at 8pm. They arranged passage for the Levys and chartered a private plan to be ready to depart for Monaco as soon as the Levys arrived in Paris. Somehow David and I still made our flight to Bermuda.

As a result of our success with the Kelly wedding entourage, I found myself arranging travel plans for General David Sarnoff, the chairman and CEO of NBC. By this time, I also had a good number of major corporate accounts, including Christian Dior, McCann Erickson Advertising Agency, RCA, and Colgate Palmolive Company.

In the 1940-s and 1950's, McCann Erickson was one of the largest advertising agencies in the world. Their headquarters were in New York, and they became one of my best clients. McCann executives frequently flew to their west coast office and usually requested the TWA Flight # 1, which carried berths. On one of those flights, we booked a senior vice president who was scheduled to be in Los Angeles the next morning for an important meeting. He asked if we could make arrangements for him to pre-board the airplane. In those days, planes pulled up to the departure gate an hour or so before the scheduled flight time, and of course I complied. He arrived at the gate at Idlewild, tired not only because of the late hour and his long day at work, but also he'd had a few drinks during the evening. TWA pre-boarded our client, who climbed into his berth, closed the curtains, and fell into a deep sleep. Somewhat later, the other passengers boarded the plane, but as the plane taxied out to the runway, the captain detected a mechanical problem and returned to the gate. The passengers were discharged and the plane was taken to the hangar. Since my conked-out friend had pre-boarded, the flight attendants apparently were not aware he was in the berth and that allowed him to sleep on peacefully unaware of what was going on around him. In the morning, he woke to find himself alone on the plane. He looked at his watch, saw it was 8am California time, got up, and dressed quickly. He rushed down the aisle of the empty plane and, when he got to the door, was astonished to find he was in the hangar. He called to the mechanics, "Please bring a ramp and get me out of here, I am due in downtown Los Angeles in a few minutes." The mechanics split their sides laughing as one said, "Man, you're going to be really late for that appointment, you're still at Idlewild."

One very interesting client was Harry Karl, the shoe magnate, who was married on and off to the beautiful actress Marie McDonald. Harry had been born in New York's Hell's Kitchen. In his early years, however, he was adopted by the Karl family, which later founded the Karl Shoe Company. The company had expanded into a nationwide organization under Harry's direction and he became a very wealthy Hollywood socialite and spent money accordingly. For example, one day he came into the office after just having purchased a Rolls Royce and asked that I have it shipped by airfreight to the coast that very day. He wanted it there for a party the next evening. I asked him if he had any idea of what this would cost and Harry responded by simply laughing, "Evelyn, don't bother me with the details."

His relationship with Marie was stormy, and the couple finally divorced. Soon thereafter, they reconciled and Harry called to ask me to book them to Paris, where they wished to be remarried. I contacted Max Boulet, the famous director of the George V Hotel, where they would be staying. He said it would

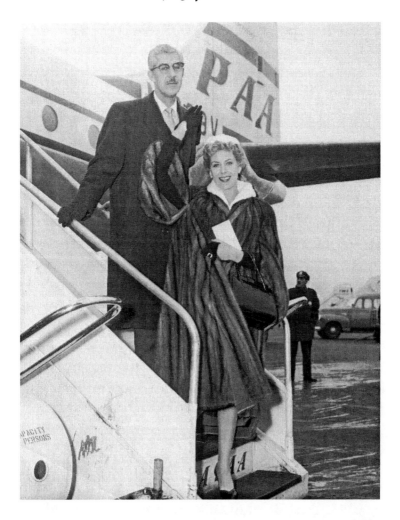

The famous actress, Marie McDonald, and Harry Karl
enroute to Paris for their disastrous second wedding.

be almost impossible to make arrangements for the
marriage at such a short notice. I left the matter in
Max's hands, telling him that money was no object
and that if bribes would smooth the way, we'd pay
them. Max handled the problem with ease, but un-

fortunately, soon after their remarriage, they once again became embroiled in one of their famous brawls. Harry left the hotel for Orly airport, where he planned on boarding Pan Am's evening flight to New York. To his surprise, when he stepped out of the limousine, he was greeted by several gendarmes who demanded in no uncertain terms that he accompany them to the airport police headquarters. After he left the hotel, Marie had called the Paris police and told them that Harry was smuggling stolen jewels out of the country. Harry was held for several hours while the police scientifically X-rayed every part of his anatomy. When the police decided he was clean, they apologized and allowed him to board a later Air France flight.

Dave and I went to Harry's apartment the following day and heard the whole story. He was still enraged making his description of what happened absolutely hysterical, especially when related with Harry's famous dry sense of humor. Nonetheless, he picked up his phone, called his lawyer, and told him to file for divorce once again.

Several years later, Harry married Debbie Reynolds. Unknown to her, his business was in deep trouble. Dan Bordett, his director of international operations and a very dear friend of ours, had tried to warn Harry that new competition, strict regulations, and high tariffs on imported shoes, were causing market loss and might force the company into bankruptcy, but Harry simply could not accept the idea that the well was running dry. He continued to live the way he had always done, and allowed Debbie to invest an enormous amount of money in the floundering company. Eventually she divorced him, his company went under, and he was forced to live out his later years in the home of his daughter.

Helen Hayes became another dear friend after we began to handle some of her many travel arrangements. The first lady of the theater was the most unflappable and courteous of travelers, much like the role she played in the movie "Airplane". One day, she was due to arrive early in the morning aboard an Italian ocean liner. She was bringing with her a new Mercedes Benz that she had bought in Europe. I went to her cabin, where she was waiting patiently for her son, James MacArthur, the "Hawaii 5-0" actor. I suggested that we remain in the cabin since it would take several hours before the cars would be on the pier. I had asked the stevedore to let us know when the car would be available to her.

The hours passed, and we still had no word. I went down to the pier to find out what the problem was, and was told that all of the cars had been off-loaded. They had failed to board her car, meaning it was still on the dock at Genoa. Since there are no guards on a pier once a ship sails, I imagine what had become of her beautiful automobile. With great trepidation, I went back to her cabin to tell her the bad news and was shocked by her tranquil acceptance of the news. She simply asked if I would let her know when the car finally arrived, hopefully on the next sailing. I thought how different the situation would have been if this had happened to one of our more volatile clients.

Most of the travel arrangements we handled for Helen out of New York were to London, Los Angeles, and Cuernavaca, Mexico. By coincidence, David's uncle, Dr. Douglas Edwards, who was a long time resident of Cuernavaca, had died. David and I were responsible to disposing of his home, and Helen turned out to be very helpful to us during this trying time. Since we were going to get rid of many furnishings in the house, I called Helen about the orphanage that I knew she supported in Cuernavaca. An American priest, Father Wasson, had started this orphanage, where at the time, about 100 orphans lived. After talking to Helen, we called Father Wasson and told him that if he would come by with a large truck and some sturdy young men, he could have an enormous amount of home furnishings. We had labeled the furniture we would be shipping back home, so when the boys arrived, we told them anything that was not labeled was theirs. They were like kids turned loose in a candy store as they loaded bedroom, kitchen, and living room furniture, blankets, pillows, and other essentials that would prove to be luxuries at the orphanage. Many years later, we met Father Wasson in Chicago and we were very sorry to hear that he had been forced to sell all of this furniture for very little money in order to buy bread. Today, this orphanage has a branch in Mexico City and is one of the most respected orphanages in Mexico.

Joe DiMaggio was one of our most pleasant clients. He and his dear friend, ticket broker George Solitaire, took frequent trips to Bermuda. He was always polite and calm, even if there was a problem. Everyone in our office competed to take his call when the operator announced he was on the line. Unfortunately, after he married Marilyn Monroe, her studio handled all their travel arrangements.

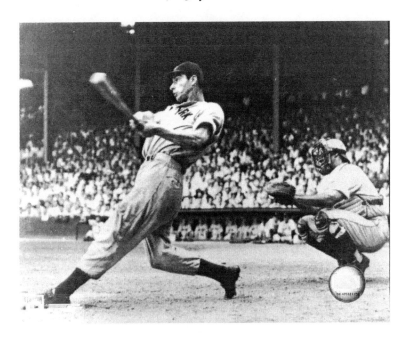

One of our favorite clients, "Gentleman Joe" DiMaggio.

In 1999, Joe came to Chicago to accept an award and I attended the dinner. He was seated at a table with his colleagues, and had given specific instructions not to be disturbed since he was not feeling well. I decided to take a chance, walked up behind him, and waited for a lull in the conversation so I could whisper, "What does the name George Solitaire mean to you?" He turned around with a big grin and said, "How the hell would you know George Solitaire?" He then recognized me, and we spent the next few minutes talking about his old friend, now deceased. It was the only time he laughed all evening. He was obviously quite ill. He departed the next morning for New York where he was being honored, then went to Miami, where he entered the hospital and died soon thereafter. Despite recently published unflattering rumors about his disposition, I always felt that "Gentleman Joe" was truly that.

In contrast, Michael Todd, who was married to Elizabeth Taylor at that time, was quite a different character. He was always in a hurry, very abrupt and quite volatile. He often chartered private planes for his travel needs, but we had a serious problem collecting payments from him. I never knew if it was because he was short of cash, or just didn't pay attention to details, but since we were a small agency, we couldn't afford to carry slow paying clients and we eventually had to sever the connection.

Both the nature of the travel business and the temperament of some of our clients made our business a high-tension affair. One of our worst days happened when we lost Burt Parks en route to Atlantic City to emcee the Miss America Pageant. About an hour before the telecast was to start, the office phones were ringing madly with people looking for him. I had chartered a private plane to take him from New York to Atlantic City, and according to our schedule, he should have arrive there at least two hours before he was due to sing "A Pretty Girl is Like A Melody." In those days, communications with private planes was far from sophisticated, and despite our hysterical efforts, we could not locate the aircraft. Finally, about five minutes before airtime, Burt Parks came running into the pageant. Apparently, our "Wrong Way Corrigan" pilot had circled Philadelphia for quite a long time trying to figure out how to get to Atlantic City. Fortunately, Mr. Parks had his tuxedo on board with him and was able to dress on the plane. When he finally landed, the waiting limousine whisked him off to the auditorium just in time. Sadly, we never received his business again, but I can hardly blame him after what we put him through.

Another dimension of my travel career began one day when my husband and I were walking down 5th Avenue and ran into a friend of David's, Tom O'Neil of the General Tires family and, at that time, owner of WOR, Channel 9, in New York. In conversation, he mentioned that WOR was considering a travel talk show and asked if I might be interested since I had considerable experience in that field. I agreed to give it a try.

The show was titled, "It's Fun to Travel" and was slotted to air on Sunday evenings at 9pm. We decided that the theme of the show would be peace through travel – the importance of the interchange of people towards world peace. This was a brilliant idea because it made it very easy for us to attract guests such as United Nations delegates, visiting foreign dignitaries, Washington politicians, and traveling celebrities. This enhanced our potential for attracting advertisers and resulted in the station increasing show time to 5 ½ hours per week at 2:30pm plus the Sunday night show.

Keep in mind in those days television shows were live and therefore if you boohooed, you did so in front of your entire audience, which made for some hilarious moments. On one occasion, I was going to interview Eleanor Roosevelt. She arrived at the station about 30 minutes before show time, and after we chatted for a bit, she asked if she might go over to the corner and sit down for a brief respite. Within minutes she was sound asleep despite the turmoil around her in the studio. We had to awaken her just before we were going on the air. She explained that with her hectic schedule, she was able to refresh herself

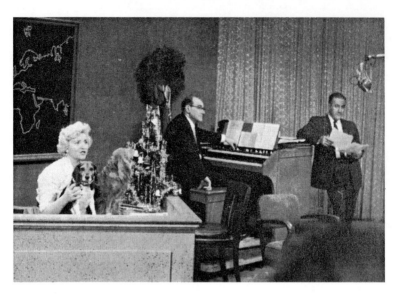

Sadie and Suzy visiting me on the set taping "It's Fun to Travel".

throughout the day with these frequent catnaps. Although I was nervous interviewing a woman of such renown, the interview was going quite well until our beagle dog, Wee Willy, who I had brought to the station that day, managed to get loose in the studio. At that point, he had discovered a rat, which was apparently directly behind our set. He was barking as only beagles can and running back and forth creating a tremendous commotion. Despite the noise and disruption, Mrs. Roosevelt sat quietly and endeavored to carry on a conversation as though all was well. Finally, Wee Willy was captured and taken out of the studio. When we finished, Mrs. Roosevelt laughed heartily and asked if she could meet the dog that had added such excitement to our show.

Another most interesting guest was Jawaharlal

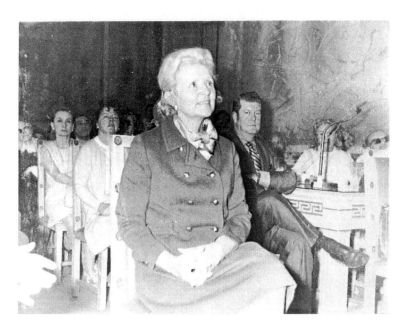

I received the keys to the city of Athens, Greece.

Nehru, the prime minister of India. He gave me such an insight into life in India that I was delighted, in later years, to visit this wonderful country on several occasions. Nehru presented me with an award from the Indian government for our efforts to promote world peace through my show. During the two years I hosted the show, we also received awards from Italy and Greece for our contributions to this worth cause.

One humorous episode occurred when Ford introduced the now famous Edsel and donated one to us for the purpose of bringing our guests to and from the studio. The Edsel had already received some very negative publicity, which the company was trying to counteract. The car arrived with the "It's Fun to Travel" logo painted prominently across the entire

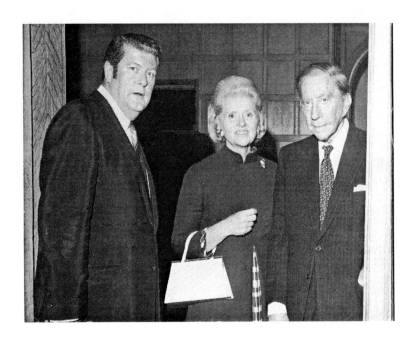

David and I visitng J. Paul Getty at his estate in Surrey, England.

side of the vehicle. One day, en route to the station, the car stopped in the middle lane at 42nd and Broadway during a peak traffic hour. Panic prevailed as the driver was unable to restart the motor despite his frantic efforts. By this time, traffic was stalled for blocks and adding to the stress of the situation, a photographer from one of the New York newspapers came along and photographed this hilarious scene of the Edsel, with our logo, being towed away to the great amusement of the gathering crowds. Needless to say, this was not the kind of publicity Ford was striving for, and after several more malfunctions, we returned the Edsel to the company with our compliments.

In the summer of 1960, David was asked to open a

Chicago office of his advertising agency, Fuller Smith & Ross, Inc. I sold my agency and ended my affiliation with "It's Fun to Travel." Actually, I was happy to sell the agency and move to Chicago. Both David and I decided that I would never go into business again.

For things past, thanks. For things to come . . . . YES!

Chapter Five

*I*n 1960, we moved back to Chicago and here again my life took on many new dimensions. Through Joan Crawford's friend, Edie Davis, mother of Nancy Reagan, I began a long-time involvement with volunteer charity work, which was not only rewarding but which brought me back to being more concerned for the disenfranchised. My introduction to Edie and Loyal Davis opened so many doors for me that I shall always be grateful.

We moved to Chicago in the month of July. David came out a few weeks earlier, and I arrived by train accompanied by our two dogs, Sadie and Suzy. A dear friend of ours, Bud Jacks, was then operating the Executive House Hotel, located directly on the Chicago River, and we chose to reside there temporarily until we found permanent housing. This was a glorious introduction to Chicago. From our terrace, we could watch the famous bridges being raised and lowered to allow the passage of larger boats, which were en route from the Chicago River to Lake Michigan. David was busy setting up his new office in the Wrigley Building, while I enjoyed this wonderful opportunity by using these lazy summer days to reacquaint myself with this wonderful city. I was also delighted since I would now be closer to my family who lived in northern Wisconsin.

In Chicago, Joan Crawford continued her kindness to me. When she learned we were moving, she arranged an introduction to Dr. and Mrs. Loyal Davis, Nancy Reagan's parents. She also contacted other Chicago friends she thought we would enjoy meeting. Her efforts made the move much more pleasant.

Since David and I had already decided that I had no interest in reentering the travel agency business, I planned to devote some of my time to volunteer work. However, my planning did not evolve quite the way I had expected, because shortly after our arrival in Chicago, I was introduced to Mary Brooks, who was then the Republican National Chairwoman and the official hostess of the 1960 Republican Convention that was set to take place in Chicago. She asked me if I would be interested in assisting her with the arrangements for the "Great Lady Fashion Show Luncheon", an important event that was to take place at the convention. I agreed, thinking that it would not require a large commitment, leaving me free to search for a new home and get settled. Little did I know that I would be devoting 20 to 30 hours per week in preparation for a major luncheon where the "cast" would

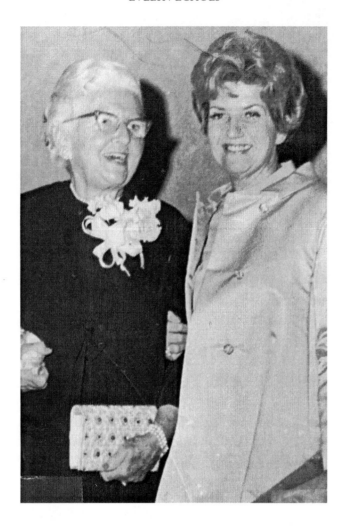

The great Edie Davis, Nancy Reagan's mother, with columnist Peg Zwecker.

include the wives of three senators, three Congressional Representatives, three governors, two cabinet members and one ambassador, all wearing copies of the inaugural ball gowns of former first ladies. Baroness Von Langendorff had arranged with the

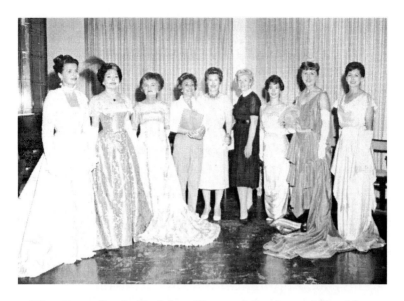

The Great Lady Fashion Show with wives of President Eisenhower's cabinet wearing copies of the former first ladies' inaugural gowns.

Smithsonian Institute to have the gowns duplicated for this celebration.

As coordinator of the event, I was responsible for negotiations at the Chicago Hilton Hotel and the dozens of problems that seemed to evolve on a daily basis. The day of the event was indeed utter chaos as the ladies were to appear on the Dave Garroway *Today Show* at 7am, which necessitated our getting them up and dressed in voluminous ball gowns by 6:30am. At the last minute, one of the cabinet wives, Mrs. Everett Dirksen, became ill. Desperate for a stand-in, we called Senator Baker's room at 5:30am to ask if the Senator's wife, who was Dirksen's daughter, could possibly take her mother's place. She readily agreed, but we had one very serious problem. The gown that she was set to wear was approximately a size 18 to 20 while Mrs. Baker wore a size 10 or 12. We finally got her pinned into the dress and on stage, where she was cautioned not to move a muscle during the telecast for fear of the dress falling apart and exposing the Senator's wife to a live audience. No one was happier than Dave Garroway, the host of the production, when the crew announced we were off the air. Since First Lady Mamie Eisenhower and Mrs. Richard Nixon, wife of the Vice President, were the guests of honor at the luncheon, we had some security problems. But, all in all, the event was enormously successful and certainly the most publicized social event of the 1960 Republican National Convention.

Shortly thereafter, when I had barely begun to unwind and get settled into our new apartment, I received a phone call from Edie Davis, Nancy Reagan's mother, and close friend of Joan Crawford's. Joan had called her saying that I was new to the city and suggested that she take me in hand. Mrs. Davis asked if I would accompany her to a meeting that morning since she had been in an accident and needed a little assistance. I walked to her apartment and off we went to a board meeting of the Mental Health Association of Greater Chicago. We were hardly seated when Edie shocked me by announcing to the board that we now have a new board member, Evelyn Echols. This was typical of Edie's modus operandi. She had not asked for a vote, nor had she consulted me; she simply decided I would be a good addition to the board. Everyone agreed and during the course of the meeting, Russell Baird, the president of the association, made the announcement that the $ 100,000 note he

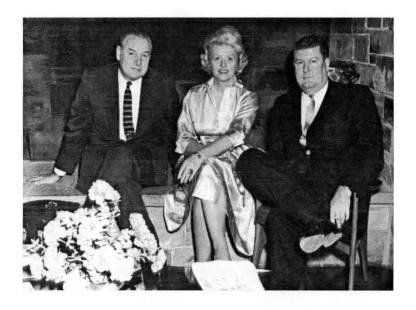

*Enjoying an evening with Governor Winthrop Rockefeller
at his Arkansas ranch, Winrock.*

had personally signed was now due at the bank and that the association had no money. I went back home and called Joan Crawford and I relayed the seriousness of the situation, which she had inadvertently gotten me into. I suggested that if she were to bring a group of her colleagues to Chicago for a gala event, we might be able to raise the necessary funds to pay off the note. She readily agreed, thrusting me into another major responsibility.

The Mental Health Association of Greater Chicago did not have a very prestigious board at this time, so Edie and I had to put together a committee to work on what would prove to be, thanks to Joan, an incredibly successful fundraising effort for the association. Generating publicity for the event was a primary con-

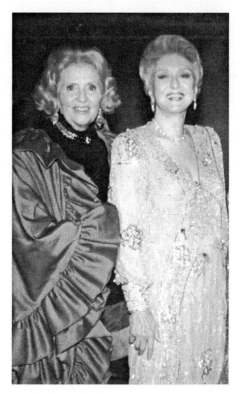

Celeste Holm attending Chicago's Mental Health Ball.

cern and would be the deciding factor in dollars raised. Mrs. Winthrop Rockefeller, wife of the Governor of Arkansas and, at that time, President of the National Association of Mental Health, had become a very good friend of mine. I decided that it would be most advantageous if she would host a weekend at their famous farm, Winrock, located near Little Rock, Arkansas, for our committee and members of the press. After some gentle persuasion, she and the governor agreed. Edie then solicited some of Chicago's major corporations to provide their private planes to fly this group to Winrock. The result of this weekend

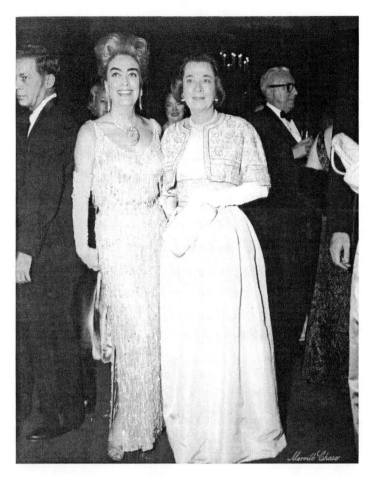

Joan Crawford with Mrs. Barry Goldwater at the Mental Health Ball.

generated enormous press coverage, and the event was practically sold out before our invitations were in the mail. Thanks to Joan's efforts, 20 major stars of that era came to Chicago, including Cesar Romero, Cliff Robertson and Dina Merrill, Mr. and Mrs. Robert Cummings, John Forsythe, Sebastian Cabot, Virginia Graham, Dorothy Kilgallen, Johnny Ray and

Celeste Holm. The event netted well over $ 100,000 which, in those days, was unprecedented. It made Russell Baird a very happy man.

I continued working with the Mental Health Association of Greater Chicago and with the National Association of Mental Health for many years. As a matter of fact, on the day President Kennedy was assassinated, I was in Washington receiving an award for my work on the National Association. I was on my way to the airport when the driver was notified of the President's death. For the next eight hours, National Airport was completely closed down. Thousands of people were walking around the airport in a complete state of shock; some sobbing, others sitting silently reading prayer books. Fortunately for me, a very dear and long time family friend, Father O'Shaughnessy appeared. He was also on his way to Chicago and was a great solace to me during those trying hours. It was only after the President's body arrived at Andrews Air Force Base that National Airport was allowed to function again.

Working with Edie proved to be a revelation. She was a remarkable woman – an old soap opera queen, who had a wonderful sense of humor and told risqué stories, which did not meet with the approval of her husband, Dr. Loyal Davis, a noted neurosurgeon. Edie loved people. If we were taking a walk around the neighborhood, every doorman in the area would come out to greet her. She not only knew their names, but the names of their wives and children and would spend a good deal of time chatting with these individuals.

One early rainy morning, I was on my way to church

and passed a building where someone had been dis-
possessed. Their meager possessions were scattered
on the sidewalk in what was now a very heavy down-
pour. I entered the building where the telephone
operator informed me that an elderly woman was the
owner of this sad collection and she had no idea where
she had gone. I turned around, went home, and called
Edie. Within an hour, she had awakened the "powers
to be" in Chicago, including the Mayor and Senator
Percy, who was spending the weekend in Chicago, and
the publishers of the three major newspapers, *the
Chicago Tribune, the Sun-Times,* and *the Daily News.*
Much to the chagrin of the building owners, photog-
raphers were gathered, shooting pictures of the now
saturated furnishings and the building with the address prominently displayed. Monday's papers all carried the story on the front page, and we were able to
locate the woman, who the Catholic Charities were
taking care of at this point. Edie followed through
until the woman was comfortable ensconced in a
modest apartment. Very often Edie and Loyal would
take underprivileged children to Cubs ball games.
They were involved in many charitable causes, which
they rarely discussed. She had many friends, yet a good
number of detractors, due in part, I believe, to the
fact that Edie said whatever was on her mind and was
completely unabashed about expressing an unpopu-
lar opinion.

Years later, when Ronald Reagan was running for
the Presidency, Edie would read every word written
about him. If she didn't approve, she would dash into
David's office unannounced and demand that he call
the New York office and have them cancel all adver-

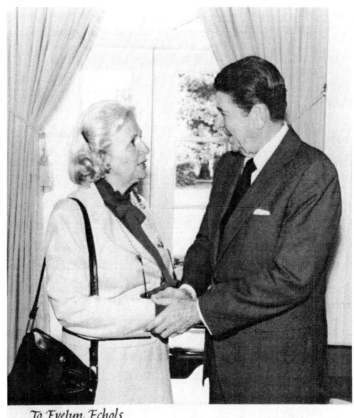

To Evelyn Echols
With best wishes,
Ronald Reagan

*Being appointed by President Reagan to the President's
Advisory Committee on Women's Business Ownership.*

tising contracts with the offending publications. Dave
had to repeatedly tell her that this was utterly impossible, but she never took no for an answer quietly or
graciously.

After Ronnie became President, I was appointed
to serve on the President's Business Women's Advisory Council, on the recommendation of Nancy. The
chairperson of our committee was Bay Buchanan, the

sister of Pat Buchanan. After we became better acquainted, she told me that they had had hundreds of requests from senators and other VIP's recommending their friends for an appointment on this committee, but when they came to mine and Nancy Reagan's name was on it, everyone automatically agreed that they would not touch this one.

We met at the White House approximately 6 to 8 times that year, and it was always an exhilarating experience. I loved going down to the employees' dining room, listening to the gossip at nearby tables. The President held a luncheon for us early on and asked each of us to tell him something about ourselves. I told him I was a protégé of his mother-in-law, Edie Davis, and he went on to relate a story, which was perfectly characteristic of Edie. He and Nancy were arriving in Chicago by Super Chief Train from California with an enormous amount of baggage. The porter entered their car and advised them that the Red Cap Porters were on strike and none would be available upon their arrival. He continued that he was at a loss as to how they would unload the voluminous amount of luggage. Nancy said, "Let's not worry about that. Mother will take care of it." Sure enough as the train pulled in, there stood Edie surrounded by four Red Caps, probably telling them a risqué story.

Our committee was designated to keep the President advised on how many of the problems women faced could be resolved. I believe that our final report to him was meaningful.

Imagine my delight when I picked up my mail one morning and found an invitation from the White House to attend a State Dinner honoring the Grand Duke and Duchess of Luxembourg. Since most of

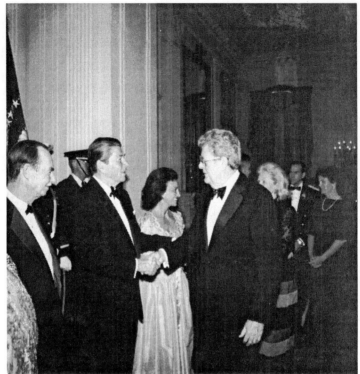

*To Evelyn and David Echols
With best wishes,*

Ronald Reagan

*David going through the White House receiving line at
the State Dinner honoring Their Royal Highnesses, the
Grand Duke and Duchess of Luxembourg.*

those dinners are limited to approximately 100
people, you can imagine the pressure from politicians and party bigwigs for these coveted invitations.

As we drove up to the White House and I was escorted by one of the military staff, I was for the first
time, truly awed by the full impact and power of the
Presidency.

Guests had gathered in the Grand Foyer and the military band struck up "Hail to the Chief". President and Mrs. Reagan were accompanied by the Grand Duke and Duchess of Luxembourg. It was such a dramatic moment that it brought tears to my eyes.

I'll always remember when I met with Nancy Reagan in the receiving line. I said, "I can't believe I'm here." She responded, "You're here because I wanted you here."

We then adjourned to the elegant State Dining Room where we enjoyed a magnificent dinner served on the new china that Nancy had just purchased for the White House. We had the pleasure of being seated with Ann Roosevelt, Chief of Protocol, and her husband, who regaled us with many fascinating stories of the goings-on in Washington. Mr. and Mrs. Henry Winkler were also at our table adding to the hilarity of the evening.

After this elaborate dinner, we proceeded back into the Foyer for dancing, led off by President and Mrs. Reagan. Shortly after midnight, they said good night to everyone and went upstairs, and this was an invitation for the guests to depart. David reminded me that evening of a remark he had made when we were leaving the Reagan's Palisades home years ago, "This guy is not stupid. With his charisma, he just might end up president one day."

I was sorry when the Davis' left Chicago and retired in Arizona, as Edie and Loyal had become extremely supportive of us and had contributed greatly to our introduction to Chicago. Years later after Loyal had passed away, I visited Edie at her home. The nurse told me that she probably would not recognize me. I entered her bedroom and was saddened by her appearance. Her eyes were closed, but as I greeted her and said my name, she suddenly rose up and said, "Well, it's a hell of a long time since I've heard from you." The old spunk was still there. She did die shortly thereafter.

For things past, thanks. For things to come . . . . YES!

Chapter Six

*H*ere is where I learned the greatest lesson in life. That's the more you give of yourself, the happier and more successful you will become.

I "cast my bread upon the waters" and was repaid a hundredfold, just as the Bible advised.

For many years, I had been praying to God for a meaningful involvement where I could render service to needy individuals. Sometimes you find the answer to your prayers not by searching but by tripping over it. I never expected to find the calling that kept me deeply involved, quite happy, and very busy for most of my life. The opportunity was given to me in the strangest way.

One evening we were at a party at a friend's house. Two of the guests were family court judges. They were discussing the problem of getting juvenile delinquents who were serving time to take an interest in learning. I made some comments to the effect that these kids were most likely school dropouts and vocational education might be a promising approach to get them involved. They might be attracted to the travel industry, in which I'd worked for many years. There is a dream quality to a travel career since it affords the opportunity to see the world and visit places one only dreams of visiting.

Like most party banter, I forgot about this conversation until one of the judges called me and asked if I'd be willing to teach a travel course at a girl's reformatory – as these institutions were called at the time. I decided to take on the challenge. I am grateful to God that I did so. It led in directions I never could have guessed at the time.

I was to teach at the House of Good Shepherd, a Roman Catholic institution run by nuns, to which first-time offenders were sent by the family court. Once there, they stayed until the age of 18. I started my first day of teaching with much trepidation. I'd never taught before and I questioned my ability to inspire these girls. Time and effort was needed to prepare for an entry-level position. Could I get them fired up enough to make it work?

A policeman met me at the gate and took me to meet Mother Helene, a remarkable, compassionate woman whom I learned to cherish. Given her schedule, I have no idea how she survived. Besides her regular daily duties, which were enough to crush a horse, she spent many a night sitting up with frightened, despondent new arrivals.

Mother Helene told me that she's chosen 15 girls for the course and took me to meet them. She introduced me and left. I noticed nervously that she locked the door behind her. Immediately, a tall young woman with a hostile attitude came up to me and said belligerently, "So, dearie, you're going to teach us the travel business? Now, you tell me, could you travel from Chicago to New York to Los Angeles and back to Chicago with only one nickel in your pocket? Could you, huh?" I said I probably couldn't do that. "Well, I did!" she sneered, and allowed as to how she thought she might be able to teach me the travel business.

Harriet was the leader of the pack, no doubt about that. And she was clearly going to be trouble. I was more encouraged by the attitude of some of the others. I told them that a wonderful world awaited them if they'd apply themselves and learn what they could about this industry, which always needs young people and doesn't require a college degree to get started. The other girls were intrigued. Harriet was not. In fact, she persistently disrupted the class. I got the feeling that she'd signed up for the course merely to avoid after-school chores.

I checked on Harriet's background. She'd been arrested several times, but she was highly charismatic and always managed to convince the authorities that she was innocent. That's why she's been eligible for the House of Good Shepherd – she had no record. I've often thought how lucky it was that she wasn't sent to a state reformatory. If she had been, she would have been lost. She seemed prone to trouble and thoroughly enjoyed conflict. With her nasty attitude, she undoubtedly would have spent a good deal of time being disciplined by prison guards who would not have been as understanding as Mother Helene and her staff.

The girls were a real challenge because I never knew what to expect. On my fourth visit, a policeman met me at the door and took me to the superintendent's office. The policeman asked me if I was aware that I was not allowed to bring indelible ink into a penal institution. I hadn't known that, and I admitted to having several bottles of ink in my file cabinet. They told me the girls had broken into the cabinet, stolen the ink, and used it to tattoo themselves. The authorities were not pleased with me.

When I went back to the classroom, I noticed they were all wearing shirts with sleeves and slacks. Most of them were giggling. They were waiting to see how I would handle the situation. I told them that they might not find this so funny when they went applying for work, that employers didn't look favorable on body art, and that it was extremely expensive to have it medically removed. I then refused to discuss it further. They then looked like a group of whipped puppies. They had been looking forward to a more heated discussion.

There were days when I had to be especially careful in how I handled them. I usually brought them small treats on these days and tried to encourage them with small compliments or awards for special efforts. They would always ask for chocolate, which I only brought on rare occasions since I felt they were hyper enough. I substituted cookies and nuts, which were always most welcome.

I realized quickly that I couldn't develop this program all by myself. I asked for and got help from friends at American Express, Cunard Steamship Line, Pan American World Airways, and TWA. Maxwell

Coker, who was then manager of the American Express office in Chicago, was one of the first to address the class. His background was in theater, and he had spent many years in England. The girls found his British accent enthralling. He had a great sense of humor. He called me after his first lecture, greatly amused, saying that this was the first time he'd given a lecture when every eye was on his trouser fly.

I got personally involved with many of my students. I found I could empathize with them, and we became good friends. At least 10 of them were really very bright. Many were at the House of Good Shepherd because they were runaways. Many of them had been abused as children – often incestuous rape at an early age. Several had turned to prostitution to support themselves. Trying to give them a solid sense of self-worth was our greatest challenge. I gathered clothes from my friends for them, and Mother Helene very sensibly allowed us to do makeup demonstrations.

The girls were also my greatest critics. I never went to the House of Good Shepherd without having my hair done or not dressing in a way that I thought they might like. Sometimes they'd approve, and sometimes I'd hear comments like "Ye gods, where did you get that?" We tried to teach them to dress in conservative business clothes once they found jobs. But sometimes after a girl found a position, I'd get a call from her employer saying that she had arrived at work in bright red stockings or a tight miniskirt – long before the mini became trendy.

We had nearly completed our first course without any major crises. Until one morning, at about 2am, the doorman of the apartment building where my husband and I lived woke us up with a phone call, saying that three young women were down in the lobby asking for me. I asked him to put one of them on the phone, and sure enough, it was three runaways from the House of Good Shepherd. At my request, the reluctant doorman escorted the three ragamuffins to our door, carrying their clothes in paper bags. He was astonished when I told them to come in. They'd been sleeping in a car for several days. They were filthy and hadn't eaten in 24 hours. I sent them off to the bathroom to wash up while I made a huge pan of scrambled eggs. Dave and I sat and watched as they demolished all the food in sight, including two loaves of bread.

The next step was to get them to agree to go back to the institution before the police caught up with them. I was worried that the House of Good Shepherd might refuse to take them back, and that they'd be sent to a state reformatory, where conditions were horrifying. I put the youngest one to bed on our sofa and called a friend of ours in the building. She agreed to let the other two stay in her apartment until morning. I wanted them to get some rest before we decided on our next move. After lengthy negotiations, the girls finally agreed to go back to the House of Good Shepherd if we would go with them, which we did. Due to Mother Helen's kindness, the incident went unreported and didn't affect their records.

At the end of the year, the class was due to graduate. I felt I should do something really special for this occasion, since this was probably the first time any of them had actually applied herself to education. I went to see Pat Patterson, then chairman of United Airlines.

I told him United should take the class up on a one
or two hour flight over Chicago and serve them lunch
on board. We'd present their diplomas during the
flight. It took a little strong-arming, but Mr. Patterson
finally agreed.

Then there was the problem of outfitting the girls
for the occasion. The Marshall Field's store and hair-
dressers from Elizabeth Arden contributed the clothes
and services. It was a very presentable group that took
off for the airport that morning. When we arrived at
the airport, I was astonished to find the media present.
Mr. Patterson had advised his company's public relations department of the event, and the PR people had
spread the word. Representatives from the Associated
Press, NBC, CBS, WGN, and Time magazine boarded
the plane with us, as did several judges from family
court. Better still, the famous singer Patty Page had
called and asked if she could come along. The girls
were ecstatic to be in her presence. They had a gloriously exciting day, giving the judges quite a hard time,
of course. There was no question; the flight strength-
ened their determination to find careers in travel and
tourism.

Even Harriet. Her attitude had improved little by
little during the course. She seemed less tough and
hostile, more cooperative. Toward the end of her stay
at the House of Good Shepherd, I found out where
some of her attitude had come from. Harriet had a
beautiful figure, but a huge disfigured nose marred
her face. After some thought, I asked her if she'd like
it if I could arrange plastic surgery for her. This tough,
strong, aggressive girl, who'd never displayed any
emotion except anger, broke down sobbing.

Through her tears, she told me that from the moment she'd entered first grade, her classmates had yanked her nose and teased her unmercifully.

Well, now I had a commitment that had to be met. I got in touch with Dr. Ira Tresley, a noted plastic surgeon, and explained the case. I told him jokingly, "I need a free nose job. Otherwise, I'll go out and campaign for socialized medicine!" He laughed and said I probably would. He asked me to bring Harriet to his office. He examined her and told her he'd do the surgery. I took her to the hospital the night before her surgery and stayed with her until she was sedated. She was so frightened that I thought she might run away if she got the chance.

The operation was a complete success. A week after surgery, Dr. Tresley carefully removed her bandages, gently applied a touch of makeup to cover the bruises, and handed her a mirror. She looked at her new nose, started to laugh wildly, and then broke into heart-rending tears. Dr. Tresley had to sedate her before we left.

We'd arranged for the teachers of the course, Mother Helene, and some of Harriet's friends to meet us at a nearby restaurant for Harriet's coming-out party. As we walked down the street, she kept looking at her profile in store windows, saying, "I can't believe this is me!" The group brought her appropriate gifts of nosegays and decorative handkerchiefs. From that day on, her personality changed. She became more cheerful, less argumentative, and even began to take an interest in the other girl's problems, something she had never done before.

After graduation, we faced a new challenge.

Harriet was one of the first girls to be released and she could easily go either way: straight or back to her previous life. We had to find her a job in a hurry. My darling husband came to my rescue again, agreeing to employ Harriet to handle travel arrangements for corporate executives in his ad agency. No one, except for the office manager, knew anything about her background. Dave kept me informed regularly about Harriet's progress. She was doing very well – always punctual, pleasant, and willing to take on any assignment. The only problem was that she seemed shy and antisocial, refusing all invitations to go to lunch with other employees. I called her and asked her to stop by our apartment, and asked her what the problem was. "Who knows how to eat in a restaurant?" she answered. This was startling to me. Who would have thought of this? But, of course, she had never in her life sat down to a meal with linens on the table.

Dave and I decided that we should invite her to dinner at our house on several occasions, which proved helpful. But we made a mistake when we asked her to a cocktail party. She drank too much and got sick and we had to take her home. I later invited her out to an upscale restaurant for lunch. By this time, she felt self-assured and comfortable. Thereafter, she began to accept invitations from co-workers to meet socially.

However, her old life kept catching up with her. Former friends would wait for her to leave the office and try to sell her drugs. The strain was starting to take its toll on her. One day, she stopped by the apartment unannounced, pale and obviously in terrible turmoil. She pulled up a chair to the window, sat down with her back to me, and said, "Mrs. Echols, you have done for me all you're ever going to do until I tell you about my background."

For the next hour, she talked about how she had lived after she left home at the age of 13. It was not a pretty story: prostitution, car thefts, pilfering anything she could in order to live. By the time she was finished, she was in tears. She got up from her chair and said, "I guess you'll never want to see me again." I put my arms around her and told her that I felt just the same about her as I always had – in fact, I appreciated her all the more, knowing what she'd been through and how far she had risen from the past. I made her lunch and sent her back to the office. From that day, she seemed to bloom.

I was delighted when Harriet agreed to give the keynote speech for the graduating class at the House of Good Shepherd the year after her own graduation. Dr. Tresley also took part in the ceremony, as did Eunice Shriver (President Kennedy's sister) and members of the travel industry. To Dave's amazement, he learned that Harriet had enrolled in a marketing course at Loyola University and was going to class with seasoned marketers. Dave worried that the course would be too advanced for her. He offered to make other arrangements with the university. She refused his intervention and went on to graduate.

Harriet was doing so well and then disaster struck. She was out on her first date with a young man, a newspaper representative who called on Dave's agency. As they were walking down Rush Street on a Sunday afternoon, they passed a group of prostitutes on a street corner. The girls recognized Harriet and ran over to greet her. Her date walked away. Again, Dave saved the situation by arranging to transfer Harriet to the agency's New York office, Fuller, Smith & Ross. When she arrived in New York, she called me and said, "Mrs. Echols, that's the first time I've ever walked through an airport when the police didn't have me in hand-cuffs."

Harriet did well in New York and eventually married into a large, delightful family that loved and cherished her for the first time in her life. We kept close touch for several years. But then I began to see I was, for her, a reminder of the old dark years. I told her that I thought it would be best for us to break off our relationship, but that I would always be there for her if she needed me. She agreed, and we parted friends. I've never heard from her since.

Shortly after my first group was released from the House of Good Shepherd, Dave got a phone call asking him to make sure that I stayed home on the morning of Mother's Day. Since I usually went to church that day, I couldn't understand why Dave kept insisting that I attend a later service – until the doorbell rang. Standing there were six of my former students. They gave me the most beautiful jade necklace from Bonwit Teller – much too expensive! They had also written a poem for me. I realized that I was now their "other mother"—something that touched me beyond words.

I had other wonderful experiences with my girls after they left the institution. With help from my colleagues, we were able to place them all. At least 10 of the original 15 went on to become successes. A few years ago, I attended a reception held by a major airline. During the evening, a woman who I'd noticed had been watching me intently all evening came over, touched my arm, and guided me to a quiet spot. There, she confided that she'd been in my class at the House of Good Shepherd. She is now in a managerial position at the airline. Of course, I was delighted to see her again.

It wasn't all perfection though. I was deeply disappointed when one of my protégés, Mildred, whom we'd placed with American Express, disappeared from the office, taking several airline tickets. She had issued them for travel from Chicago to Los Angeles for herself and another person. She had also written another one and had convinced the airline to allow her to cash this ticket in – something she could not do today. I was concerned that this would have such a negative effect on American Express, I asked Catholic Charities to cover the losses, which they did.

In 1978, I picked up my mail and found a letter with a return name and address that I didn't recognize. It was from Mildred. Inside was a check for $ 1,500 and a note that said how sorry she was for what she had done to me. It had taken her years to save up the money to repay her obligation. She had married and was raising two children. She worked for a doctor and lived in a nearby suburb. Mildred asked me to come visit her, and we had a joyous reunion. We sent the $ 1,500 check to Catholic Charities to repay them.

One Christmas Eve, Dave and I spent the entire evening down at the detention home for young delinquents, trying to get one of the girl's younger brothers released to our custody for the holidays. It was well past midnight when the judge, whom we'd called at home, finally agreed, as long as the boy stayed with us until he was returned to the penal facility. Looking back, I think it was incidents like this that made our program successful. We worked with these young women on a one-to-one basis and put in considerable time and energy on their behalf. They knew we would go to the wall for them, for any legitimate purpose. That knowledge, that slowly growing trust, kept them with us through the program. There were so many times in their rehabilitation when we could have lost them.

I spent a good deal of time at the detention home with Margo, the social worker from the House of Good Shepherd, as she went through the process of choosing candidates for her institution. I remember going up to the dismal quarters where these young offenders were housed and finding, to my horror, that abused babies and small children were also being held there until social workers could find foster homes for them. I cannot begin to describe how pitiful these little ones were. They would hang on me, crying desperately and begging me not to leave. It broke my heart. I knew then that I had to get involved in fighting for better conditions for these innocent victims. We finally succeeded, but as usual in dealing with bureaucracy, it took some battling.

After two years, Mother Helene left the House of Good Shepherd, and for some inexplicable reason, our program was cancelled. I was extremely upset by this decision, especially when I found that the girls were taking ballet lessons in the time slot our course had occupied. A Roman Catholic orphanage approached me and asked if I would like to conduct the course on their premises, since they had a good number of teenagers who might benefit from the experience. We introduced the course and continued to teach it for several years until the orphanage closed. Again, we turned out highly qualified young people who were able to find jobs in our industry as soon as they were 18 and on their own.

A whole new career was opening up for me. United Airlines' publicity of the House of Good Shepherd graduating class had led to a flood of inquiries from people looking to pursue careers in travel. But there were no programs for them and training incoming employees was a major problem in the industry. Clearly, there was a crying need for a travel school. My husband and I decided to explore the feasibility of setting up such a school. I went to New York and proposed our idea to the corporate executives with whom I had worked for years when I owned my own travel agency there.

My first call was to C. R. Smith, a friend of my husband's and chairman of American Airlines. I described the program we had in mind and told him that we were certain it would succeed if professionals taught the courses. I was delighted with his reaction. American Airlines would help me write the curriculum and would teach the air section for the program. I met with equal success when I visited Cunard Steamship Co., American Express Travel Services, Holland American Cruise Co., and Pan American World Airways. Harvey Olsen, president of the famous travel agency in Chicago, also became one of my main supports.

I flew back to Chicago in early August. I still had

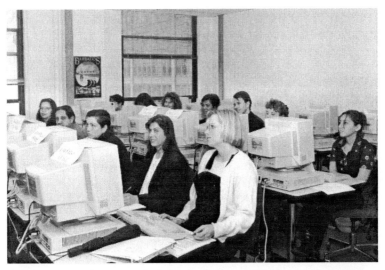

Students at the Echols International Travel & Hotel School, 1997.

no real promotional materials, but I managed to entice 15 students into enrolling in our first class, starting September 23, 1962. From that starting point, it was clear sailing for a long, long time – 35 years. We opened branches in San Francisco and Washington, D.C. The Echols International Travel and Hotel School in Chicago graduated more than 12,000 students, many of them inner city young people whom we helped with scholarships.

Dr. Hazel Steward, principal of Tilden High School, sent me a good number of students for training. When this particular group was about to graduate, I asked the Sheraton Hotel to host a luncheon for them, their parents, and potential industry employers. They served up a wonderful spread of hamburgers, hot dogs, ice cream and soft drinks. The Bottomless Closet, an organization that collects used clothing from businesswomen, outfitted the girls, who were beautifully turned out and well coordinated. We managed to round up good clothes for our young men from one of Chicago's major department stores, Carson Pirie Scott. The travel industry delighted me by sending representatives from at least 15 major travel and hotel companies. Some of the students were hired on the spot; others were given business cards and asked to call for an interview. The Sheraton Hotel itself snatched up our valedictorian, whose speech was genuinely inspirational.

It delights me even now when I hear from my former students. Recently, I was passing the American Eagle Airline check-in counter at O'Hare Airport and I noticed three African-American airline representatives, two of them checking in passengers and one working the gate. When they spotted me, they ran out to greet me. It was such a joy to see how proud they were, and how professional they looked in their crisp uniforms. Helen, the young woman working the gate, said, smiling widely, "Mrs. Echols, you have no idea how important I am here! Do you realize no one can board this aircraft unless I let them?"

When I was sitting in St. Patrick's Cathedral in New York a few months ago, two women leaned over the back of my pew, asking, "Aren't you Evelyn Echols?" I hadn't seen them since 1964 when they'd been students of mine at the orphanage. After the service was over, we went across the street for coffee. I learned that they were both working for a major New York hotel.

Hardly a month goes by that I don't hear from one or another of my former students – something that gives me a wonderful sense of pride. Not one has ever called me because he or she needed help. It's always a good-news story. It humbles me that my help has made a difference to these people.

"Cast your bread upon the water, and after a time, you may find it again," the Bible tells us. That's what I found. My small initial investment paid me back a thousand-fold, in ways I never could have expected and that have enriched and brightened my life. I can only thank God for this accidental calling. And that I do.

For things past, thanks. For things to come . . . . YES!

Chapter Seven

The older I get, the more I appreciate the need for the interchange of people if we are to have world peace. We must all learn to appreciate other cultures and what better way to learn this lesson than through world travel.

Our travels throughout the world have greatly contributed to David and my happiness, memories, and our concept of life. Although every trip added another dimension to our lives, there are three that are most frequently in my memory: Russia, India, and Italy.

RUSSIA

In 1961, David and I were invited to join the American Society of Travel Agents on a trip to Russia. We flew from Chicago to Frankfurt, Germany on Scandinavian Airlines. From there, we had the enviable experience of flying to Moscow on the Russian airline Aeroflot. The service on Aeroflot was quite different from what we are accustomed to on flights as Americans. The first problem was that the carpet was not attached to the floor of the cabin, causing me to trip on my way to the rest room. No food was served, and the disgruntled staff seemed totally unimpressed that travel agents could produce great numbers of tourists and that our accompanying members of the press would be writing about their travel experience. On arrival at Moscow's airport, they scrutinized our luggage for a minimum of two hours and primarily seemed interested in any books or magazines, which they confiscated.

By the time we arrived at the hotel and checked in, we felt like a group of starving refugees as we dashed to the dining room. Here we encountered another great surprise, because we were so late, the staff had simply put out large containers of boiled potatoes on the tables and left. This was to be our dinner, and upon inquiry, we found there were no restaurants open in the vicinity. How about candy bars or snacks? Nyet. We did find a few nuts in the bar and that was it.

Needless to say, the sheets and blankets in our room were not exactly what you would find in a Four Seasons Hotel. The following day, Intourist, our official hosts, notified us that we would be picked up and taken on a tour at 8am. Although we were warned to travel only with an Intourist guide, Dave suggested it would be more fun if we took off on our own after the tourist buses departed. We walked a short distance to the railroad station and spent several hours watching the commuters arrive. Some immediately knew we were from America and were most anxious to

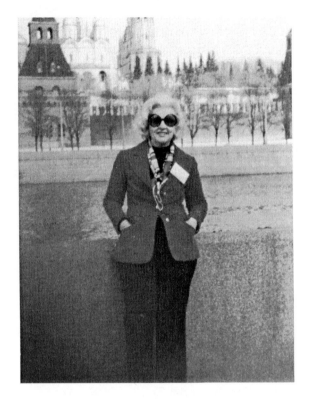

At the Kremlin during that eventful Russian trip.

speak with us. Several made inquiries about how to get visas to come to the United States. We also consumed a huge breakfast from street vendors – and survived. We then decided to take a trip on the famous Russian subway, which was a wonderful experience. This was rather daring since we had no idea where we were going, but felt that if we only traveled a short distance, we would have no problem finding our way back home. As we got to the station, we could not believe how steep and endless the escalator seemed as we descended to the platform. To our surprise, we discovered that the train tunnels were extremely clean and decorated with beautiful murals. We traveled to the next station, disembarked, crossed over to the other side and returned without difficulty. We felt we were being followed but couldn't be sure of this.

That night we were guests of the government at an official reception. Never before have I seen such enormous containers of caviar. This delicious delicacy was gobbled up unceremoniously, accompanied by wonderful large snifters of iced vodka. We were greeted by a good number of government officials, most of whom spoke perfect English. I was dancing with a gentleman who kept trying to converse with me in Russian. A friend of mine, Carol Abrioux, danced by and said, "For God's sake, Evelyn, don't step on his toes. He's the head of the KGB." With this my dancing partner cracked up laughing, having understood every word she said. From then on, our conversation and our dancing were much livelier. He even tried to teach me some Russian folk dancing, and eventually he did admit that he was, indeed, the director of the KGB.

After another day of exploration, we attended the ballet, a glorious experience. We attended a magnificent performance of "Romeo and Juliet". I have always had great respect for the Russian people because throughout their history, no matter how impoverished they were, they always supported the arts. Thanks to one of our traveling companions, who at the time was director of the Italian Tourist Office in Chicago, we had one glorious Italian meal after returning from the ballet. He had brought all of the ingredients to make pasta and invited us to supper at the Italian Embassy. No food ever tasted as good nor was as welcome as this delicious meal.

We returned to the hotel rather late but after saying goodnight to everyone, David thought it would be a fantastic idea to go our and walk through the Kremlin. We had an eerie feeling as we left the hotel that we were being followed. When we arrived on the grounds of the Kremlin, it was still brilliantly lit. Although there was not a sound or sign of any other person, we still were under the impression of being followed and hoped if we were arrested, our American passports would be honored. We spent at least two hours strolling through this historical majestic site, discussing its history, and the fate of many people who had lived and worked here over the centuries. This was indeed the most impressive part of our sojourn.

The following day, we went to Leningrad, now known again as St. Petersburg. Founded in 1703, the city has the aura of a great imperial capital. As we walked along the Neva River, it was hard to imagine the horror the city had experienced during World War II, when it was under siege for 900 days and its citizens were dying from exposure and starvation. Our first impression of Leningrad was positive since all the people we encountered were extremely friendly. Many spoke English and seemed anxious to communicate with us as we passed them in the streets.

A day in the Hermitage was the highlight of our Leningrad experience. This world famous gallery was built in 1763 as a secluded retreat for Catherine the Great. She moved her art collection into the Hermitage, and over the next century and a half many more additions were made. Today, the Hermitage has 150 rooms filled with the world's greatest paintings and sculptures. For example, in one room alone, there are 27 Rembrandts. The four-room suite at the top level overlooking Palace Square houses paintings by Renoir, Matisse, and Gauguin in an incredibly beautiful setting. The trouble with the Hermitage is that there is no climate control, and temperature fluctuations have led to a tragic deterioration of many of the paintings.

After our two-day visit to Leningrad, we returned to Moscow before heading home. This trip left such an imprint in my memory that I now enjoy a greater appreciation for Russian music, dance and art.

INDIA

"If India grabs you, you will never be the same," my dear friend, Norman Ross, told me before my first trip to that country. India did grab me, and it has held on ever since, but it didn't start out that way.

My husband and I journeyed to India in the early 1970's. We arrived at the airport in Bombay one early evening. As we drove to the Taj Hotel, we first witnessed the squalor of the people who lived under the bridges we passed by. Every day, the bodies of the people who died the night before are picked up off the street and piled into carts. In the early morning, Mother Teresa's nuns rescue some of the dying people and care for them until they die. I was violently ill from our observations by the time we arrived at the Taj Hotel, as was David, and had we not been

guests of the Indian Tourist Bureau, I sincerely believe we would have called the airline and booked
immediate flights home.

What made the immense poverty around us all the
more jarring was the drastic contrast with the other
magnificent sights in Bombay: sacred cattle walking
in the streets, snake charmers, elephants, old jalop-
ies so overloaded with people they looked like cir-
cus acts, Rolls Royce's carrying golden-robed maha-
rajas and beautiful women in exotic saris entering the
Taj Hotel. It didn't take long for us to discover the
beauty and dignity of the many impoverished people
we encountered during our first few days in India.
The hotel had arranged for us to visit the temple of
Mumba Devi, a goddess revered by the local
Mahastian people and for whom the city of Bombay
was renamed, Mumbai, in 1996. When we arrived in
the early evening, I was immediate enthralled. As we
lit a candle and joined the procession leading to the
shrine, I glanced at the tired, withered faces that were
everywhere around me, and was amazed at how patiently and quietly everyone waited for their turn to
enter the shrine, where they would bow their heads
and pray reverently for several minutes before depos-
iting their candle on the altar. I thought of how different it was from the people who often jostled one
another on their way to receive communion at
churches in the United States.

In Indian, among Hindus, the caste system deter-
mines the social status and occupations of every indi-
vidual. The caste system consists of four categories.
Brahmins are the priests, scholars and teachers;
ksatriyas are the warriors and rulers; *vaisyas* are the

professionals, merchants, and artisans; and the *sudras* are the laborers and servants. About 15 percent of the Indian population, which was 906 million in 1998, are known as *untouchables* and are outside the caste system. The only positions available for these unfortunate souls are the most undesirable jobs, such as cleaning toilets. Although the government supplies certain jobs for these individuals, they are greatly discriminated against. They are banned from many Hindu temples and aren't even allowed to draw water from certain wells. Many people believe that if they come in direct contact with an *untouchable*, they will be contaminated and tainted. According to Hindu beliefs, these positions within the caste system are destiny, the result of karma. Their attitude is that individuals must accept their lot and not try to change how the cycle of life, death and rebirth turns out. Therefore, many *untouchables* strive to make a living from begging.

We encountered some of these *untouchables* on our last day in Bombay. We invited the young concierge at our hotel, Josephina, who had taken such good care of us, to join us for lunch. Since the restaurant she recommended was only a block away from the hotel, Dave suggested that we walk. Josephina was apprehensive about this because of the hundreds of beggars who would be pleading for money along the way. In the United States, we are used to violent street crime, but it is rare in India. Beggars don't carry guns or knives, and since these people are never violent, we opted to walk.

In the vast crowds surrounding us, we observed one young boy whose histrionics were incredible. His piercing eyes and beautiful expression were most captivating as he clasped his hand and pleaded with David. I wished I could have packed him up and brought him home with me, dirt and all. David asked Josephina if there was any way he could possible donate to the boy's cause, but she said the others would probably attack the boy if David were to hand him anything. Just as we were about to reach the restaurant and he realized his efforts were going to go unrewarded, this street smart kid, whom we thought did not speak English, suddenly yelled out, "Well, then f*** you, mister!" At this, Dave and I laughed uproariously. Dave said, "I'm giving this kid some money, and I bet he's smart enough to get through this crowd intact." He was so smitten with this child that he cleaned out all the rupees in his pocket, the equivalent of $ 15, which our hero grabbed and stuffed in his pants. He then sprinted off before anyone could possibly get a hold of him.

At the time, I was hosting a travel television show in the United States and Indian government officials had invited us to explore the country as their guests. We left Bombay and headed to Jaipur and New Delhi. As we headed into the countryside, we came upon a group of six women, and although they were obviously impoverished, they were all beautifully clad in an array of homemade, brightly colored saris. Each carried a large jug of water on her head, but maintained perfect posture and walked gracefully, which thoroughly amazed us as they carried out the arduous task of transporting the water at least 5 to 10 miles, a daily ritual for survival due to the arid conditions of the area. At every lake and pond, we would see women like these and others who were washing their family laundry and laying it out in the sun to dry, making a carpet of wondrous color along the shores.

After spending a week traveling from Bombay to Jaipur to New Delhi, David and I were exhausted when we got to our hotel, but I was about to face something I had never before experienced. Immediately after checking in, my old friend and famous designer in New York, Bena Ramada, was there to greet us. She decided I looked fatigued and needed some relaxation. She suggested I go to the hotel health spa for a yoga lesson and later introduced me to the yoga teacher, a beautiful 80-year old woman, named Madam Rabaldi. She took me by the hand and quietly spoke to me in her cultured Indian English accent and I felt that I was in the presence of an angel. For the next five days, she taught me the basics of yoga and maintaining inner balance. Since those five days with Madam Rabaldi over 35 years ago, my daily routine has started with a 30-minute yoga stretch period, which I think, in many ways contributes to my well being today. Thank you, Madame Rabaldi.

The second leg of our trip took us from New Delhi to Agra to visit the Taj Mahal. En route via automobile, we encountered throngs of people who were walking, riding in buses, on elephants, and in carts pulled by cattle. Luckily our driver spoke many different Indian languages and was able to glean that this mass of humanity was headed to see the Prime Minister, Indira Gandhi, who was visiting a new oil well facility. These joyful people, many of whom were walking distances of 20 to 30 miles in the broiling 100 degree sunlight, were waving excitedly at us and

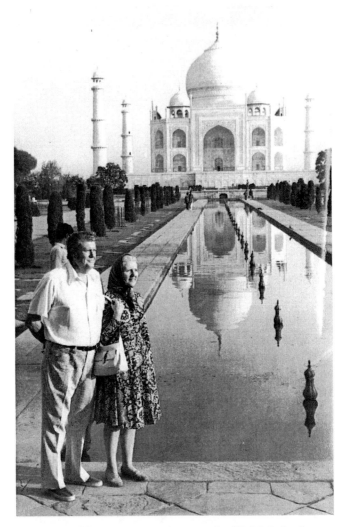

Our glorious morning at the Taj Mahal.

getting out of the way to make room for our car. I was amazed by their politeness and how quiet such a large crowd could be, which was later reported to be almost one million people.

Once we arrived at the location where Gandhi

would be appearing, we stepped out of the car and our driver walked ahead of us. Then an incredible thing happened. This massive crowd, who had expended such enormous effort to get here, cleared a path for us. It was like Moses parting the Red Sea. We were very embarrassed by this since seeing the Premier was much more important to these people that it was to us. When we refused to move forward, they insisted and we ended up right in front of Gandhi. A few times, I thought I would collapse from the intense heat, and I believe I only survived because of the low humidity. Mrs. Gandhi arrived around 20 minutes late and spoke for 45 minutes. Fortunately, our driver had given me his chauffeur's hat and David was wearing a sun hat that he had purchased in New Delhi. As we were leaving, a good number of people in the audience spoke to us and wished us happiness and a full life.

We continued on to Agra and the next morning, thanks to the courtesy of the Indian Tourist Office, we were allowed entrance into the Taj Mahal at 7am, three hours before it was open to the public. No experience in my life will ever compare to the time we spent alone in this monument to love. Shah Jahan was the father of 13 children, and built the Taj Mahal in memory of his beloved wife, Mumtaz Mahal, who died in 1631. Construction of the Taj required 20,000 workers and 18 years to complete. Since the sun was just beginning to rise over the Taj, we were able to see how the marble, inlayed with precious jewels, changed colors and moods with each hour. I'm sorry that we were not able to also see it under the light of a full moon because I understand this too is a spectacular sight. At the sacred spot, where the tomb lies, I sat down on the floor, overwhelmed by beauty. Shah Jahan was later overthrown by his son and forced to live out the rest of his life jailed in a tower with a view of the Taj, and his dreams of building a duplicate in black were left unfulfilled.

David and I wandered in different directions, both of us so completely absorbed in what we were seeing that there was no need to converse. I walked out on the grounds and looked down the Yamuna River where a man appeared, disrobed to his shorts and immersed himself up to his chest in this filthy water. There he stood facing east and saying his morning prayers for at least an hour. Ten o'clock arrived quickly, and David joined me out on the grounds where we sat quietly in reverence for our surroundings. As the gates opened and hundreds of people began to flood onto the premises, we said a prayer of thanks for the three hours we had spent in the presence of the most beautiful monument ever produced on this planet.

Our final destination in our adventurous trip was to Kashmir, reputed to be the garden spot of the world. However, getting there was an adventure unto itself. We boarded an Air India flight in New Delhi, and after waiting for a very long time, we were told to deplane because they forgotten to fuel it.

Happy were we that they discovered this slight error before taking off. Later when we were airborne and beginning our flight over the Himalayas in a blinding snowstorm, David handed me a daily newspaper that had a headline that read, "Air India pilots refuse to fly by instruments. They prefer to rely on their own

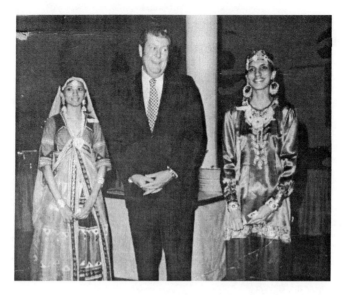

Doesn't David look bewitched?

instincts." The article went on to say that this had caused some accidents. What joyous news now that we were flying in a canyon where, when looking out the window, the gigantic white covered mountains on either side seemed to be scraping the wings of our plane. Fortunately, neither David nor I were afraid to fly, but I did notice quite a number of white knuckled passengers grabbing their airsick bags.

For well over an hour, we continued in what was a scene of magnificent beauty, despite hazardous conditions. When the pilot finally said, "We are coming in for a landing," the thought that he was not relying on technology made us somewhat apprehensive since it would be impossible for the crew to see until we were practically on the ground. They set the plane down with great aplomb, and as we were de-planing, Dave asked them to join us for a drink later, which they did. Yes, it was true, they had not made use of the instruments available to them feeling as though it would ruin their macho image.

We were taken by cab out to the houseboat we had rented for a week on a lake. The houseboats here were beautifully furnished with lovely antiques and wonderfully hand-woven rugs. There was color everywhere. Our manservant was an excellent cook and served us beautifully out on the deck. In the mornings, while we were having our breakfast, vendors would arrive, offering their wares. They would paddle out in canoes loaded with a glorious array of flowers, especially the pink lotus blossoms, which have religious significance in India. Others were selling jewelry, knick-knacks, paintings, carpets, saris, hand-woven bags, and artwork of every description.

Needless to say, we purchased much more than we had ever expected to and fortunately, the Greek Counsel General in Chicago, our friend, Nico Macridis, had told us that we could ship all of our purchases to him, thereby avoiding customs and delays. Incidentally, he was very shocked to find weeks later that all of his offices were loaded with packages from India.

Watching the sun come up over the Himalayas in the morning and set in the west in the evening from this magnificent setting was an incredible event in our lives. We left there with a sense of peace. It is so sad that the ongoing war between Pakistan and India prevents others from having this wondrous experience nowadays.

We drove back through the countryside to New Delhi, boarded a plane, and flew home. As our plane circled over the Himalayas, I felt the grasp of India that my friend had referred to. I knew that my experiences of the past three weeks had left such an indelible impression on me that I was not the same person I was before the trip.

ITALY

Italy, especially Tuscany, has always been my favorite place on earth. David always said if we were going to Bermuda, I would somehow find a way to route us home by way of Rome. One very special night, we came out of a nightclub at about midnight and discovered we were directly across from the Forum. It was a beautiful moonlit night and we decided rather than going directly to the hotel, we would take a leisurely walk through the famous ruins located between the Palatine and Capitoline Hills. The Forum was now completely unoccupied, not a soul in the area. As we walked silently to the Curia, we visualized senators and famous orators pleading their cases, and Julius Caesar making his impassioned speech before he was assassinated. We spent two hours mesmerized by the history we were imagining and finally emerged through the Arch of Titus. David and I agreed over the years that this was one of our most awesome experiences.

Friends in Chicago had recommended a driver in Rome to us. The following day, Bruno took us on a tour of the Coliseum and other places of interest. He was a walking encyclopedia, not only of Rome, but also of the entire country. Of course, he took us to wonderful intimate Italian restaurants where the pasta was incomparable. The following morning, Bruno took us to the Vatican, but due to Pope John Paul's heavy schedule, a private audience could not be arranged for us. However, thanks to Bruno's many contacts, on entering St. Peter's Square, Bruno was able to maneuver us through the crowd with the assistance of one of the Vatican priests. We were seated in the first row as the Pope left his study window and proceeded to walk around the entire square. It was obvious Bruno had connections because His Holiness came directly to us and spent two or three minutes talking to us. As he held our hands, we felt the presence of a truly holy man. We were surprised when some beautiful pictures of the meeting were delivered to us at the hotel, compliments of the Vatican.

However, the truly incredible was yet to come. On the third day, when Bruno picked us up, he said he was taking us back to the Vatican. We could not understand as we had spent several hours touring the area after the Pope had completed Mass. En route we took on another passenger, an official from the Vatican. We drove through the back entrance of the Vatican, entered a building and ascended a series of stairs. Suddenly we realized we were in the Pope's private quarters. Bruno and his friend showed us the Pope's dressing area and opened all the closets to display his vestments and the cabinet in which he kept his gifts for special visitors. Bruno said, "What would you like to have?" Dave said, "We don't want a damn thing. Just get us out of here before the Pope walks in in his shorts!" Bruno assured us the Pope never got up until a certain time, but at David's insistence, we then scampered out of these sacred quarters as

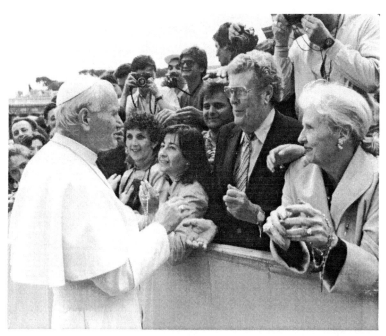

Being greeted by the Pope at the Vatican in 1980.

quickly as we could. We could now understand why His Holiness, the previous day, had turned to Bruno as he was leaving us and queried, "Bruno, what am I going to do with you?"

Bruno was now going to drive us through Tuscany and into Florence. This is my most favorite area in the entire world and we enjoyed three days exploring the Tuscan Hills. One particular day we spent in Assisi, we were to celebrate Mass at the Basilica of St. Francis, but had arrived a little too early, so we stopped at a nearby confectionery and bought two huge ice cream cones of semifreddi chocolate plus a large box of incredible candy. Now we were sitting on a curb at 8am pigging out, much to the amusement of the natives. After a beautiful mass at the Basilica, we de-

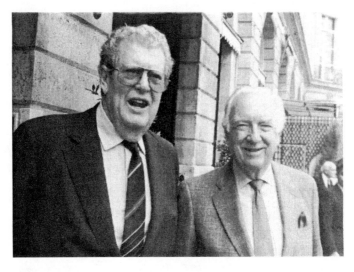

David and Walter Cronkite attending the 100ᵗʰ Anniversary of the International Herald Tribune in Paris.

scended the stairs to where St. Francis is buried. There, a gentleman wearing a tuxedo came to us and said his daughter was to be married in the small chapel and he invited us to observe the wedding. It was a beautiful affair, with four splendid Italian tenors who sang the Mass. After the service, we were also invited to attend the reception, but felt we should be on our way to Florence.

Florence, to me, is the representation of the Garden of Eden. I love the ambiance, the architecture, the ancient sights, museums, music, people and unsurpassable food. Since I was still associated with the travel industry, we were guests of the Grand Hotel and they made their penthouse suite available to us, which had a terrace that overlooked the entire city of Florence and the Arno River. Naturally, we spent a good deal of time shopping and taking ad-

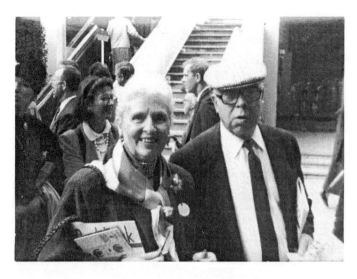

With Art Buchwald, attending the 100th Anniversary of the International Herald Tribune in Paris.

vantage of the beautiful arts, crafts, leather goods, and silk scarves that are available in hundreds of shops throughout the city. We spent four days in this beautiful spot before proceeding to Venice.

We had said goodbye to Bruno and David bravely decided he would drive the rest of the way. We rented a Fiat, which unfortunately broke down on one of the busiest highways in Italy. We were stalled, for what seemed like several hours, amid catcalls and insults from irate commuters. Several had tried to push us off to the side of the road but to no avail. Finally, a Fiat truck happened to be passing and saw our dilemma. We could not believe what was happening when the two mechanics lifted the entire front end of our car, shook it up and down several times, set it down, and away we went.

We arrived in Venice and were again hosted by

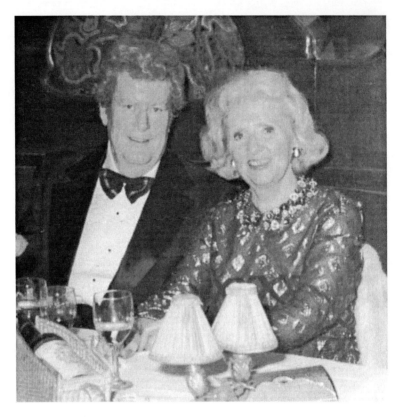

Maxim's in Paris, New Year's Eve, 1956.

the Gritti Palace Hotel, which is located on the canal.
Here we spent a wondrous three days touring one of
our favorite cities. We enjoyed many hours of oper-
atic music and people watching in St. Mark's Square.
On the last day, we took a motorboat out to the elegant Cipriani Hotel as guests of the manager, Mr.
Resconi. As we were having lunch on the terrace on
this gloriously sunny day, he asked us when we were
planning to leave. We told him we would be leaving
later in the afternoon for Milan but were sorry that
the Orient Express did not board in Venice. He hap-

pily replied, "Oh, I don't know about that, we own the Orient Express." He immediately left the table to make reservations for us. What an impressive way to exit Italy! The trip was much too short, but we were extremely grateful for this accommodation. We arrived in Milan just in time to transfer to the airport for our trip back to the United States.

David and I cherished the memories of our many travel experiences and what we learned from them. It enriched the life that we shared together all the more and helped us appreciate our last few years together.

For things past, thanks. For things to come . . . . YES!

Chapter Eight

With David's death, my life changed dramatically. I was now flying on one wing. In thinking back, it was amazing to me that I was able to function at all. I kept thinking of Dave's final admonition to me, "I'm going to give you three months to get back to life and I'll be watching." Thank God for the many friends who came to my rescue and the fact that I was forced to continue to work. It took much longer than three months to recover, especially with the other problems I faced, but eventually I came back to life.

In 1990, my life was to change dramatically. And if it had not been for the ever-present help of the Lord, I hesitate to think what my life would have been like for the next seven or eight years.

That year, David's doctor told him that he had a very large aneurysm in the aortic artery. The doctor went on to say that this artery could rupture at any moment, resulting in almost immediate death. On returning home from the hospital, David said, in his usual optimistic fashion, that we should not worry about this problem because doctors were not gods and he planned on being around for some time.

He went back to work as a consultant at Bozell Advertising and continued to teach his highly successful New Product Lab course, which he had introduced, at the University of Chicago's Graduate School of Business. He loved his involvement with the students and was happy about contributions he had had been making at the university for the past 15 years.

So our lifestyle didn't change much, except that now I began to slowly turn my responsibilities at the travel school over to a newly hired manager. I made up my mind that when David called and said "Hey, how about lunch?" or if he was coming home early, that I would always be there.

From the outset, I realized that the general manager I had selected would eventually get us into trouble. My employees, particularly my treasured Chief Financial Officer, Ron Tully, began warning me that this manager was not up to the job. Ron recommended that I sell the school immediately. This I refused to do, confident that when David died, I would be able to rebuild the school to its former stature. We had enjoyed the enviable reputation of being "the best travel school in America for 32 years" according to Holiday Magazine. Although I was very aware of the problems at the travel school, I never let David know my concerns.

Because of his optimistic attitude, life went on much as it had during the past 40 wonderful years.

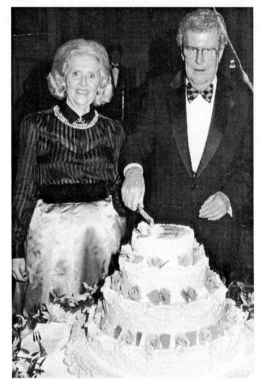

David and I at my 75th Birthday Party!

We found our greatest happiness in time spent together. I believe that because of the cloud that hung over us, we treasured those moments more than any other time in our lives. My daily prayer was that David would be at home when the end came and not away on business. Due to the fact that a ruptured aorta is extremely painful, I prayed that I would be there to get him to the hospital, allowing doctors to ease his pain during the last hours of his life.

We had purchased a wonderful condominium in the 1950's, the first one offered on Sanibel Island in Florida. For a cost of $ 59,000, this proved to be a special haven for us where we spent one to two

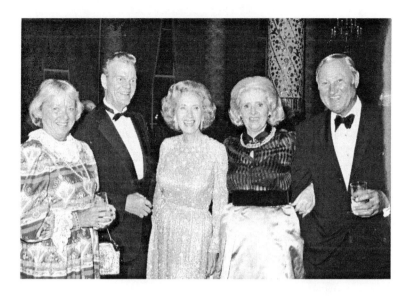

Martha Mlakar, Paul and Angel Harvey, Chuck Mlakar, and I at my 75th Birthday party.

months every year. It was located right on the Gulf of Mexico, and since we usually went to the island in November and December and then again in March, we avoided the crowds of vacationers who descended on the island during the winter months. Early in the morning as the sun was just rising over the gulf, we would take a two-mile walk down to the lighthouse accompanied by hundreds of seagulls, sandpipers, pelicans and porpoises, affording us great entertainment. We usually stopped for breakfast before our walk home and spent the rest of the day quietly on the beach.

Due to the fact that we had such busy schedules when we were in Chicago, we did not get socially involved with our neighbors, and we both appreciated the seclusion of the island. This was a period when life was completely effortless, and how glorious are the memories of those respites.

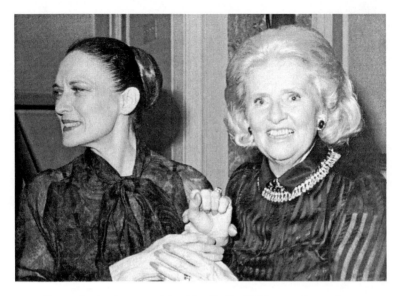

One of my dearest friends, Julie Wilson, the cabaret singer, came to Chicago for my 75th Birthday party.

David's business took him to New York on quite a regular basis and I would always accompany him since I was afraid the end might come soon and didn't want him traveling alone. New York had always been one of our favorite cities and one where we had many friends so we thoroughly enjoyed those visits.

On August 25, 1995, we took off for Wiesbaden, Germany, to celebrate David's birthday and our 44th anniversary. I had chosen this destination because, although he did not complain, I noticed that David's energy level was diminishing and the Nassaur Hof Hotel had a wonderful spa, which I thought would be beneficial to him. The spectacular pool, located on the roof, is fed by mineral waters located directly under the hotel. This location is where Napoleon brought his troops for R & R. After spending a few

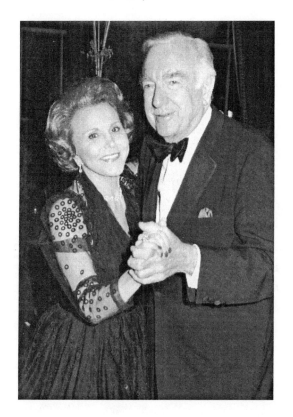

Ann Landers and Walter Cronkite enjoying a dance at my 75ᵗʰ Birthday party.

hours in the pool, we noticed that David was able to walk much longer distances.

On our anniversary, David had ordered a delicious breakfast including a small bottle of champagne. He then went to the closet and took out a large white box beautifully decorated with a pink satin bow and placed it on the bed. He presented me with a hand-written message of love that brought me to tears. Our friend, Ann Landers, once said that she would give anything to have a man look at her the way David always looked at me. Now he too was crying and as we embraced on another, although we did not voice it, we knew this might be our last anniversary together.

My tears gave way to laughter when I opened his gift – a most glamorous French lace chemise and gown, in about a size 10. As I held it up, saying, "Darling, do you truly believe I could get into this?" he said he didn't know why not. I could not believe he still saw me in that light, especially since I now weighed 160 pounds.

Reluctantly, he agreed to go back to the store and I shall always remember the look of incredible surprise on the sales lady's face when she saw the woman for whom this gentleman had made the purchase. I am sure she had assumed that some little cookie would be the recipient. As we selected an exquisite, yet more appropriately sized 14 gown, we all enjoyed a good laugh with the other clerks who had joined in the merriment. As we were leaving, we heard our sales lady say to her associates, "*War das wunderbar!*" – wasn't that beautiful!

They had agreed to deliver the package to our hotel so we made our way to the dock for the noon luncheon sailing up the Rhine. It was a gloriously sunny day, one I will always treasure. The boat was not crowded and as we enjoyed a lovely lunch with a delectable bottle of wine. We passed some of the world's most beautiful scenery. It was an awesome sight to see — centuries-old castles and miles and miles of picturesque vineyards, green forests and gorgeous flowers in every direction, as far as the eye could see. I only wish that everyone could experience this afternoon of Rhine sailing.

Exhilarated by our experience, we returned to the hotel, took a siesta, and then celebrated our anniversary in the exquisite and intimate dining room of the hotel. That night, as we retired, we agreed that this was indeed our best anniversary. Thank you, God!

After coming back to Chicago, David immediately returned to the university and set about making preparations for the forthcoming semester.

Saturday, September 9, was a gloriously sunny and bright day in Chicago. We took McDougal, our sassy yorkie, for a walk in the park and returned home around noon. We drove up to Lincoln Park and then spent the next two hours strolling through the beautiful grounds, taking time to enjoy the glorious flowerbeds and allowing Mac to chase the largest dog he could find so that he could assert his authority over them – even though they could gobble him in one bite. It always amazed us how Mac managed to frighten these animals and send them scurrying for cover.

We stopped by the zoo to watch the ever-amusing porpoises and returned home happy and invigorated. I prepared lunch and Dave opened a good bottle of cabernet wine. All seemed in divine order on this delightful day. Little did we dream that this would be our last day on earth together. David watched the Notre Dame football game and then said he was going to take a nap. I was in the kitchen when I heard him call me. I went into the bedroom and before he even spoke I knew the inevitable had happened. He was ashen and was having difficulty standing. He apparently was trying to get to the bathroom. He spoke quietly, "Darling, I'm sorry to be leaving you. The artery has ruptured."

David had lived a full, happy, fulfilling life over the past five years, but now it was over. Thinking back, I believe I did exactly what we agreed would be done on this fatal day.

He laid down on the bed and as I held him, I called 911. We had agreed that we would get him to the hospital and under no circumstances would the doctors torture him needlessly by endeavoring to save his life, but would immediately administer morphine intravenously. While we waited for the medics to arrive, we talked about the 44 years of incredibly beautiful life we shared. This was a love story that very few are ever fortunate enough to experience. Some believe it never happens. Believe me, it does. We lived for one another and thereby made one another totally happy through good times and bad. As his voice became weaker, he said that the very happiest days of his life were the times we were alone together.

The ambulance arrived and as we were admitted to the emergency room, it was fortunate that I had not only his living will but also his power of attorney. They were determined to take David up for X-rays and since our doctor was out of town, I stood alone in my determination that they would not allow him to suffer through meaningless procedures, but would mmediately begin morphine injections and leave us alone. My assertive threat of a lawsuit finally convinced everyone to do as I wished.

Our good friend, Father McLaughlin, pastor of Holy Name Cathedral, arrived and prayed with David and administered Last Rites. He also gave me wonderful words of encouragement. After Father departed, we had probably another 30 minutes before

David began to lapse into unconsciousness. At this point, he could not speak above a whisper, but he did manage to say, "You have been the most wonderful wife any man could ever hope for. I will give you three months to get back to life and this you must do. I'll be watching over you." In the last moment, he raised his head, looked directly at me, and barely whispered, "love". And then he was gone. As long as I live, those treasured moments will remain in my memory and give me great solace.

I found the medical staff to be extremely cold. I presume this is the way they are trained to be, but as most people I have spoken to agree, it is wrong. It is dehumanizing. One nurse did come in and ask if I wished to sit with David for a while. Why? He was gone. The gentle, handsome, brilliant, humorous, love of my life was no more. I simply wanted to get home, where I could be alone. Some very sympathetic volunteers took me to a cab and offered to accompany me home. However, despite the fact that I was numb with grief, I declined their offer. I spent the night praying and contemplating how my life had changed in the last several hours and pondering how I would address the many problems now facing me. How was I going to survive without David's constant care and concern? No more romantic interludes. No one to tell me how beautiful I was every day, even though I knew I was now well over 80 years old and no longer the well known model and TV personality he had married in 1951.

In the early morning hours, I gathered the strength to call our children, relatives, friends, and business associates. I spent the following days making funeral arrangements despite the fact that I was still functioning in a state of shock. The support and love of our children and our close friends sustained me during this very sad period.

It is amazing how our Creator helps us through these times of crisis because certainly on my own, I was too numb to function. Hundreds of friends, students from David's classes at the University of Chicago, people he had helped throughout his generous life, all came to pay their respect. Then it was over. The children went home to California. Relatives had said their goodbyes and I was alone again. The Moody Institute radio broadcast "Music through the night" helped me get through the long hours when sleep was impossible.

It was only after everyone had left me that I regained full consciousness. The funeral was held on a Tuesday. The very next morning I called the travel school to say I would return the following day. I knew if I were to retain my sanity, I would have to stay extremely busy. I asked that the staff not mention David's passing since I could not talk about it. Students, teachers, and staff all greeted me, showing their deep concern with kindly gestures and making it possible for me to get back to work.

What a blessing it is to be busy, having problems to solve and decisions to make for ten hours per day! What work would I have done otherwise?

Friends insisted that I accept all social invitations, which was wise. My inclination was to get into bed and pull a pillow over my head. Thank God for my many loving friends.

Around this time, I was beginning to realize how

serious the financial problems were at the school. My enrollment had fallen from 500 students a year to around 200. The school's expenses had also accelerated enormously — far outpacing income.

Both Ron Tully and my financial advisor and dear friend, John Meinert, urged me to close the school immediately, before I incurred more debt. This I refused to do because I felt I could reestablish Echols International School to its former glory, attract the number of students I had in the past and over time, recapture our losses. I worked long hours and poured most of my resources into keeping the school going. I could not let my devoted staff and the many loyal companies who had supported me over the years suffer because of my mistaken judgment.

Despite my best efforts, the situation continued to deteriorate. I simply didn't have the heart or energy to keep going. So, in 1997, I was forced to close the school.

'Tis said that God does not give you more problems that you can handle. Well, he must have had a great deal of confidence in my ability to handle adversity from 1995 to 1998.

David had died thinking he had left me financially sound, when actually I was in debt well over $500,000. I had encouraged him to let me sell our Florida condo since we were using it only occasionally, and I had invested the $250,000 selling price into the school. With Ron Tully's cooperation, I was able to make the investment without consulting David. This was very important to me because the doctors had warned me that any mental anguish could result in the artery rupturing. I had also borrowed a great amount of money from beloved friends. However, I was not too concerned because I felt that when David died, I would sell our 40-acre farm in Grayslake, IL. Since property values had increased dramatically, I was confident that I would then be able to repay my debts and still be financially sound. This was not to be.

We had, in 1996, subdivided the farm into five-acre lots and were about to close on the sale of the first one when my real estate agent called and said he had dreadful news for me. The Metra Railroad, a suburban mass transit line, ran through our property. They had a terrible accident the previous year when one of their trains hit a school bus in Fox River Grove, IL, killing a number of children. This experience so traumatized the directors of Metra that they decided that I could not sell any of the property until I installed a $300,000 railroad crossing, complete with gates and signals. Obviously, I didn't have that much to invest. Therefore, while we tried to negotiate this problem with the railroad board, I was forced to pay taxes on the property. Eventually, the bank foreclosed and I suffered an enormous loss again.

Unless I established another source of income, I would be reduced to a very bad financial state. But as often happens when one hits rock bottom, our guardian angels take over. As I was contemplating how to get back on my feet, Paul Vallas, CEO of the Chicago Public Schools, called and asked if I would be a consultant to the Chicago Board of Education, training inner city high school students to be prepared for entry level positions in the tourism industry. Since tourism and travel had been my lifetime career, I enjoyed my new role to the fullest. This position would not only enhance my income, but would keep me involved in the education of young people.

I continued my many other interests, including serving on the boards of several business and civic organizations. My feeling was that the busier I was, the less time I would have to devote to feeling sorry for myself. However, I had to face new limitations.

For things past, thanks. For things to come . . . . YES!

Chapter Nine

*J*ust when I thought things were turning for the better, I had another blow. And I began to think God had lost track of me. Macular Degeneration!

What is that? I soon found out.

However, I also discovered this was not the end of the world and once again, life goes on. At 88, I'm living a full, happy, and content life and actually wouldn't change places with anyone else. It's been a great run and I'm looking forward to some new surprising challenges. What fun!

After my husband's death, I noticed that I was having greater difficulty reading. I was frightened but refused to pay a visit to my ophthalmologist for several months, as I was sure the condition was due to grieving and would improve with time.

Finally, my concerned office staff practically forced me to call the doctor. He insisted that I come in immediately. Unfortunately, the macular on the left eye was no longer functioning either. Since I had waited so long to address this problem, it was too late for any type of successful laser surgery. My doctor spent a long period of time recommending ways to make my life more pleasant as a *legally blind person*.

Being referred to as legally blind brought reality to the whole situation. I was devastated. But on looking back, I know that this is what made me step up to the plate and decide that despite this handicap, I would go on and lead my life as I had when I had been able to see the beautiful world around me.

It seemed as though I was seeing everything through a heavy fog. I could no longer read any print less than one inch in size. I went with great trepidation to the Foundation for the Blind. The individuals there encouraged me greatly. Through them, I purchased a television set specially equipped to magnify print. By placing reading material on a plate under the TV, I could then read the highly magnified print that appeared on the screen. What a godsend!

Everyone recommended that I use a cane for fear that I would fall. This I flatly refused. I soon found that by keeping my head slightly turned I could make maximum use of my peripheral vision. I soon regained the confidence to hold my head up and maintain an erect posture. To date, my guardian angel has helped me to keep from falling in one of the many potholes I encounter on my almost daily one or two mile walks. I do have to be very careful when crossing streets so usually I wait until I determine that other pedestrians are proceeding. If no one is around and I can't read the signal, I listen to the sound of the car motors, which indicates when I would have the right of way, and say a little prayer before I step out into the street.

The necessity of working and enjoying what I do is a great advantage. Idle time is the time we are inclined to feel sorry for ourselves, so I'm delighted to have very little time for the indulgence. Although I have changed my career somewhat, I am still involved in teaching young students how to be prepared for an entry-level career in travel and hospitality. I also still feel a responsibility to contribute so I remain very active on civic boards. This benefits me because it keeps me mentally challenged and I have the feeling of gratitude, that at age 88, I'm still able to contribute to mankind.

One of the most difficult lessons I had to learn during these past few years was patience. Sometimes, it will take me five to ten minutes simply to put a plug into a socket. I found that swearing about this aggravation did not help. I soon realized that I was spending possibly one to two hours a day just looking for things – especially magnifying glasses. It took me some time before I finally learned that I must put things in the same place at all times. I started singing to myself as I put something down . "Tra la la . . . I'm putting my glasses on the kitchen counter." My memory seems better when I sing.

Learning to put makeup on by rote was a real challenge. Finally, with the help of many friends, I conquered, and from all comments, seem to be quite adept at this daily ritual. Eye makeup, especially applying eyeliner, was a real trial. My friend, who is a makeup artist, suggested that instead of trying to

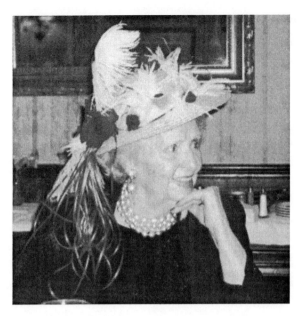

My 80th Birthday party with the Brigadiers—wearing the hilarious hat they presented me!

apply it above my lashes, I apply it below them and this proved to be a wondrous solution. I'm not good at doing my hair and still have to visit the beauty parlor on a weekly basis. One major problem is that I cannot determine color. I have gone out with one brown and one black shoe. I also have a problem with hose since I cannot tell whether or not I have a run. Before stepping out into the street, I now ask friends in my building or even my doorman to look me over and give me their okay. Yes, I still wear high heels when going out in the evening.

One special blessing is that I still have a very large contingency of younger friends. This keeps me from the situation many older people find themselves in, where they spend too much of their time going to the funerals of their friends, until they begin to feel desperately alone. Having become bored with most cocktail parties where interesting conversations seldom take place, I decided to invite six younger women to my home for dinner. I decided that they would be women who were not acquainted with one another and that the topic of conversations for the evening would be "What is the craziest experience you have ever had with a man?" Since I can no longer trust myself to cook, I simply ordered Chinese food sent in.

The evening was a huge success. We laughed uproariously over one another's bizarre experiences. They left well after midnight and the next morning were on the phone demanding that I do it again. Today, this group of 40 women calls themselves the Echols Brigadiers and we meet monthly at one another's homes. Since many of these women travel or have other obligations, the number to attend is usually about 25. The hostess chooses the subject we are to discuss and I'm blessed to see how many wonderful friendships have developed in the group. They even bought me an authentic Brigadiers hat, which I wear to all meetings.

Besides this wonderful contingent of younger friends, another thing that has kept me presentable is the care I take of myself and my appearance. It particularly disturbs me when older people stop taking care of themselves and their hygiene. I'm reminded again of Joan Crawford's advise to me years ago when she told me to be so beautifully turned out that people passing me on the street would think I'm on my way to a romantic interlude. I follow her advice everyday.

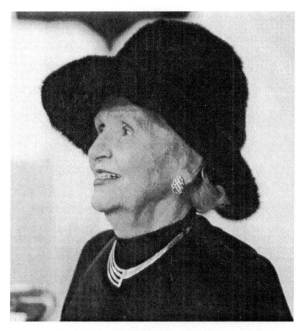

A noted lecturer once told me to always wear a hat when
speaking because it gives the audience something to look
at while you're warming up.

Another thing I believed helped me through crisis situations is that I am quite disciplined. I practice yoga every day. I find it keeps me physically agile, which is terribly important, as one gets older, and also contributes to my mental alertness. I continue to swim everyday which makes up for the fact that I'm not always able to walk along Lake Michigan or through Grant Park because of Chicago's winter weather. I have become a vegetarian and find that by never eating a large meal at one time, my heart is happier.

Today, at 88, I believe that I am the most fortunate person alive and I would not change places with anyone. I continue to serve on numerous charity boards and I love sharing my life's experiences by lecturing at universities and civic organizations. This past October I spoke to 800 students in Washington DC at the national Collegiate Entrepreneurs' Organization annual conference. Of the 46 keynote speakers, I was voted one of the top THREE speakers by the collegiate participants.

I'm still looking for new adventures. I believe you live each day to the fullest but always keep looking for the fun that awaits you in the future.

My constant prayer is that when I can no longer function on my own, that God will take me home. I also have the confidence that my beloved Dave is watching over me daily. I feel that my partnership with God has contributed so much to my life, and I hope that you too, dear reader, will come to this same conclusion.

For things past, thanks. For things to come . . . YES!

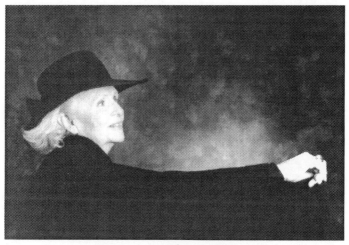

About The Author

At 88, Evelyn Echols continues to lead a very busy
social and business life.

She writes.

She lectures.

She serves on 6 charity boards.

She's still collecting awards from foreign governments
for her work in promoting "peace through travel".

She dances.

She travels.

She swims and practices yoga.

She feels that her very active life and her spiritual
guidance keep her gloriously happy.

BVG